Benchmarks:
Alternative Methods
in Toxicology

Edited by:

M. A. Mehlman

Published by:

PRINCETON SCIENTIFIC PUBLISHING CO., INC.
Princeton, New Jersey

Printed and bound in the United States of America.

PRINCETON SCIENTIFIC PUBLISHING CO., INC.
P.O. Box 2155
Princeton, New Jersey 08543
Tel.: 609/683-4750

LIBRARY OF CONGRESS CATALOG NUMBER: 88-063539 ISBN 0-911131-19-1
Cover Art: Adapted from

Benchmarks:
Alternative Methods
in Toxicology

ACKNOWLEDGEMENT TO CONTRIBUTORS

We wish to thank the following for their support of this publication:

American Cyanamid Company

The American Society for the Prevention of Cruelty to Animals,
 John F. Kullberg, President

Animal Rights International
 Henry Spira, Coordinator

Animal Welfare Institute
 Christine Stevens, President

BP America, Inc.

The Helen V. Brach Foundation

Chevron Corporation

The Coca-Cola Company

E. I. du Pont de Nemours & Co., Inc.

Exxon Corporation

The Humane Society of the United States,
 John A. Hoyt, President

The Massachusetts Society for the Prevention of Cruelty to Animals,
 Frederick J. Davis, President

National Institute of Environmental Health Sciences

R. J. R. Nabisco

PepsiCo, Inc.

Pfizer, Inc.

The Procter & Gamble Company

G. D. Searle and Co.

Shell Oil Company

Dorothy and Richard Sikora

U.S. Department of Agriculture

Palmer Wayne

We wish to express our special thanks to the U.S. Department of Agriculture for
major funding for this book.

CONTENTS

PREFACE
M. A. Mehlman 1

ACUTE TOXICITY TESTING, PUBLIC RESPONSIBILITY AND
SCIENTIFIC CHALLENGES
Gerhard Zbinden 3

METHODOLOGIES FOR INTERPRETATION OF SHORT-TERM
RESULTS WHICH MAY ALLOW REDUCTION IN THE USE OF
ANIMALS IN CARCINOGENICITY TESTING
Fanny K. Ennever and Herbert S. Rosenkranz 15

CASE, THE COMPUTER-AUTOMATED STRUCTURE EVALUATION
SYSTEM, AS AN ALTERNATIVE TO EXTENSIVE ANIMAL TESTING
Herbert S. Rosenkranz and Gilles Klopman 29

PHYSIOLOGICAL PHARMACOKINETIC MODELS: SOME
ASPECTS OF THEORY, PRACTICE, AND POTENTIAL
Richard W. D'Souza and Harold Boxenbaum 37

AN OVERVIEW OF STRUCTURE-ACTIVITY RELATIONSHIPS
AS AN ALTERNATIVE TO TESTING IN ANIMALS FOR
CARCINOGENICITY, MUTAGENICITY, DERMAL AND EYE
IRRITATION, AND ACUTE ORAL TOXICITY
Kurt Enslein 59

IN VITRO TECHNIQUES IN TERATOLOGY
George P. Daston and Robert A. D'Amato 79

IN VITRO SCREENS FROM CNS, LIVER AND KIDNEY FOR
SYSTEMIC TOXICITY
Charles A. Tyson and Neill H. Stacey 111

ACUTE OCULAR IRRITATION EVALUATION: IN VIVO AND
IN VITRO ALTERNATIVES AND MAKING THEM THE
"STANDARD" FOR TESTING
Shayne C. Gad 137

ANIMAL RIGHTS AND MODERN TOXICOLOGY
Leonard Rack and Henry Spira 193

UTILITY OF SHORT-TERM TESTS FOR GENETIC TOXICITY
David M. DeMarina, Joellen Lewtas, and Herman E. Brockman 205

SUBJECT INDEX 217

PREFACE

In recent times, alternative methods in biomedical research and safety evaluation of chemicals and compounds have come increasingly to the fore. This development represents the confluence of several factors: 1) accelerating developments in basic biologic methodology and understanding, especially *in-vitro*, 2) increasing realization of the wastefulness of such tests as the classic LD_{50} and Draize, once useful but now considered archaic, and 3) increasing insistence from the public and animal rights groups that new understandings and methodologies be pressed into the service of reducing animal use and alleviating animal suffering.

This volume, the first in a series, represents a joint effort by internationally recognized scientists from the diverse disciplines of industry, government, academia, and the animal rights movement. These papers are intended to serve as a catalyst for rapid identification, validation, and implementation of alternative methodologies. The term "alternative" can be defined as using methods which (1) Replace the use of animals, (2) Reduce the number of animals used, or (3) Refine existing procedures so that animals are subject to less pain and suffering. A fourth "R" may be added to these—Responsibility.

The "4R" principles are actively promulgated by sectors of the animal rights movement and, in particular, by one of the foremost representatives, Henry Spira, a contributor to this volume and coordinator of the coalitions to abolish the Draize and LD_{50} tests. These principles are increasingly discussed in the scientific community, and implementation is well underway particularly in the toxicology sector.

Looking ahead, we see alternatives leading to a brighter future for all. Alternatives tend to be faster, cheaper, and more predictive of toxicity of chemicals, and they can lead us to a win-win situation in which human health and the environment will be more efficiently and better protected.

ACUTE TOXICITY TESTING, PUBLIC RESPONSIBILITY AND SCIENTIFIC CHALLENGES

GERHARD ZBINDEN

Institute of Toxicology
Swiss Federal Institute of Technology and University of Zurich
Schwerzenbach, Switzerland

Knowledge of the acute toxic effects of chemicals is important for the protection of exposed humans. Since sufficient information in humans is often lacking, experiments on laboratory animals must be performed. The LD_{50} test, which requires large numbers of animals, has become the preferred procedure. It is now widely criticized on scientific and ethical grounds. This paper reviews the possibilities of using fewer animals to obtain relevant information on the acute hazards of chemical substances, but it also identifies the reasons why the traditional testing approaches cannot be changed immediately. An important problem is the practice of basing legal decisions on classification of chemicals in official lists of hazardous substances and for labeling purposes on LD_{50} values. Proposals are presented on how pain and suffering of the animals included in acute toxicity tests can be reduced. The use of in vitro systems for the evaluation of the hazardous properties of chemicals is discussed.

CONVENTIONAL APPROACHES TO ACUTE TOXICITY TESTING

Overwhelmed by a mass of chemical substances which followed in the wake of the Industrial Revolution, the primary concern of scientists was the protection of the public against acute intoxications. And even today, when the emphasis in toxicology has shifted toward the problems of chronic exposure to low levels of chemicals in the environment, increasing numbers of accidental poisonings and recurrent tragedies of mass intoxication, such as the recent disaster in Bhopal, serve as a stern reminder that the threat of acute intoxications is still a serious concern.

The situation is aggravated by an accelerating output of new chemicals. About one thousand new substances were registered daily by the Chemical Abstract Service in

1. Address correspondence to: Gerhard Zbinden, M.D., Institute of Toxicology, Swiss Federal Institute of Technology and University of Zurich, CH-8603 Schwerzenbach, Switzerland.
2. Key words: acute toxicity testing, drug interactions, hazard assessment, median lethal dose.
3. Abbreviations: LD_{50}, lethal dose 50%, median lethal dose.

1983 (Maugh, 1983), and this figure, most probably, has increased substantially by now. Although only a fraction of these new agents appears at the workplace and in the environment, the hazard of chemical accidents is increasing. Thus, the protection of the public against acute poisoning remains an important obligation of toxicologists and the public health profession.

An essential prerequisite for instituting realistic protective measures is the knowledge of the toxic properties of chemical substances. Since sufficient experience in humans is often lacking, animal experiments are used as a substitute. From the observation of small numbers of laboratory animals poisoned with large doses, considerable knowledge on symptomatology, target organs of toxicity, cause of death and reversibility of signs of intoxication can be gained. As a collateral piece of information, data on approximate lethal doses in various animal species are obtained (Zbinden and Flury-Roversi, 1981).

Although this procedure is satisfactory for the purpose of gaining general information on poisonous properties of chemicals, it lacks the precision necessary for certain objectives, particularly the standardization of highly toxic biological agents such as insulin and digitalis extracts. Therefore, an experimental method was developed to measure the median lethal dose (lethal dose 50%, LD_{50}) of a substance in comparison to a simultaneously investigated reference sample (Trevan, 1927). Briefly, groups of 5, 10 or more animals per dose and sex are treated with single doses of the test substances, ranging, if possible, from a non-toxic dose to one causing mortality of all or the majority of the subjects. The animals are observed for at least one week. The time of death is noted, and the median lethal dose (LD_{50}) is calculated, using appropriate graphic or biostatistical methods.

It is not readily understandable why the LD_{50} test, which requires large numbers of animals, became the preferred, and soon the only procedure accepted by regulatory agencies for the assessment of acute toxicity. Regardless, it is now widely used for all kinds of agents, including drugs, pesticides, industrial chemicals, even the essentially inert cosmetics and food additives, and it has found a place in every toxicological testing guideline issued by national and international regulatory bodies. Moreover, it has gained further prominence as the major test on which the official classification of hazardous chemicals is based.

SHORTCOMINGS OF THE LD_{50} TEST

In recent years the current practice of acute toxicity testing has come under attack by animal rights advocates and antivivisectionist groups. At the same time, toxicologists have criticized the procedure on scientific grounds (Zbinden, 1973; Sperling, 1976; A.B.P.I., 1977), and several reviews have dealt with these issues in detail (Zbinden and Flury-Roversi, 1981; Le Beau, 1983; Dayan et al., 1984; ECETOC, 1985). The major shortcomings of the LD_{50} test and of its application in safety testing programs are summarized in Table 1.

TABLE 1
Shortcomings of the LD$_{50}$ Test

The numerical value of the LD$_{50}$ is not a biological constant, but highly influenced by endogenous and exogenous factors.

The LD$_{50}$ test considers mortality and neglects morbidity.

The LD$_{50}$ determined in animals has little predictive value for the lethal dose in man.

Comparison of the LD$_{50}$ in newborn and mature rodents is not a reliable method for detecting special risks in human neonates.

The LD$_{50}$ does not provide a reliable basis for dose selection in repeated-dose toxicity studies.

Determination of combined LD$_{50}$ is not an acceptable method for risk assessment of drug combinations.

Comparison of LD$_{50}$ by oral and parenteral administration is a wasteful and unreliable method for assessing bioavailability.

The use of LD$_{50}$ values as a basis for classification of hazardous substances neglects many properties worthy of consideration. Moreover, various countries use different classification criteria.

In the LD$_{50}$ test, some of the animals are subjected to extreme pain and distress.

However, it must also be acknowledged that acute toxicity testing in laboratory animals is not without merits. Experience has shown that the procedure can provide useful information on signs of intoxication, target organs of toxicity and cause of death, provided that the experiments are performed by well-trained personnel, using all available techniques to monitor physical signs and pathomorphological changes of the organs (Zbinden and Flury-Roversi, 1981). Data obtained in properly performed acute toxicity studies have a high degree of predictability for many of the functional disturbances and organ lesions occurring in humans, pets, domestic and wild animals exposed accidentally to chemical substances. Thus, acute toxicity studies in laboratory animals can contribute substantial information to the overall knowledge of the hazardous properties of chemical agents.

CURRENT NOTIONS AND CONTROVERSIES

Among the vast majority of industrial, regulatory and academic scientists there is broad agreement about the utility and the shortcomings of acute toxicity tests, as they are presently performed. From the lively discussion going on in many scientific circles, societies and expert groups, it has become clear that much important information on the acute toxic hazards of chemicals can be obtained with small numbers of animals. It has also been shown that it is often not necesssary to use doses that cause mortality in a substantial number of the subjects (Tattersall, 1982). Other scientists have resumed the approaches of earlier workers (Deichmann and Le Blanc, 1943; Thompson, 1947; Deichmann and Mergard, 1948; Dixon and Mood, 1948; Weil, 1952; Brownlee et al. 1953), and have demonstrated convincingly that it is possible to determine LD$_{50}$ values with satisfactory precision, using a total of 12 animals or less (Mueller and

Kley, 1982; Schuetz and Fuchs, 1982; Lorke, 1983; Bruce, 1985). Moreover, the British Toxicology Society (1984) has issued a proposal permitting classification of hazardous chemicals with few animals and with no need for a numerical value of the LD_{50}.

In the light of these encouraging developments, the question must be asked why the conventional methods of acute toxicity testing with large numbers of animals have not been abandoned long ago. Two factors that have worked against a rapid change of current practices can be cited, the toxicological tradition and the laws controlling hazardous substances.

Toxicological Tradition. The determination of the LD_{50} has, for many years, been the most frequently performed biological test with live animals. Medicinal chemists and pharmacologists have come to rely on it for the calculation of therapeutic indexes, biostatisticians have used it to develop their concepts of the "bioassay," toxicologists took it as a point of reference, and regulatory agencies have looked at it as an indispensable part of registration dossiers (Zbinden, 1983). The following example will illustrate this point: In a recent paper, Brimblecombe and Leslie (1984) reviewed the preclinical safety studies with the H_2-blocker cimetidine and compared them with the adverse effects observed in clinical practice. Among the undesirable reactions missed in animal toxicity studies was the dangerous potentiation of dicoumarol anticoagulants, leading to episodes of bleeding in several patients.

In the preclinical safety program with cimetidine, the possibility of hazardous drug interactions was investigated carefully. As a matter of fact, interactions with as many as 29 drugs were considered. However, the traditional approach, namely a combined LD_{50} determination, was used to identify substances that might be hazardous when used together with cimetidine. Considering the mechanism of action of the dicoumarol anticoagulants, it is easily understood why such an experiment failed to recognize a potentiation of the anticoagulant effect by cimetidine. A very simple bioassay which measures the relevant response, namely prolongation of prothrombin time rather than mortality, was able to predict reliably the hazards of the drug combination (Table 2).

This fact was also belatedly acknowledged by the authors of the paper, who write: "The drug interactions now known to occur with cimetidine were not predictable using acute toxicity studies as the test procedure. This type of interaction study is widely demanded by drug regulatory bodies, but the value of results is not very obvious, especially in view of the very large numbers of animals used. It is noteworthy, for example, that the interaction with warfarin did not show up in these tests. The design and interpretation of these studies is a matter for considerable debate and it is almost certain that more complex and more specific tests. . . are appropriate for the production of enzyme induction and consequent drug interactions. There would also be a considerable saving in the use of animals."

TABLE 2
Combined Effects of Cimetidine and Warfarin in Blood Coagulation in Rats[a]

Treatment	Prothrombin time	Stypven time	Partial prothr. time
Control	15.4 ± 0.7	17.2 ± 6.3	20.5 ± 4.6
Warfarin	23.9 ± 4.7	26.0 ± 3.3	31.9 ± 2.6
Cimet. 100 mg/kg	13.6 ± 0.6	10.8 ± 0.8	21.9 ± 3.3
Warf. + Cimet. 100 mg/kg	28.2 ± 4.1	22.9 ± 3.5	34.0 ± 8.4
Warfarin	26.7 ± 4.5	35.9 ± 6.2	48.5 ± 4.5
Cimet. 200 mg/kg	15.1 ± 0.6	16.3 ± 0.6	26.3 ± 2.8
Warf. + Cimet. 200 mg/kg	$40.7 \pm 4.8**$	40.8 ± 4.6	$59.4 \pm 7.1*$

[a]Groups of 6 Sprague Dawley rats (SIV) were treated with cimetidine or equal volumes of water twice daily by gavage for 4 days. On the 4th day 0.4 mg/kg warfarin was administered orally, and blood coagulation tests were performed 20 hours later. All results are given in seconds. $*$ = statistically significant difference in comparison with rats treated with warfarin only. P 0.05, $**$ = 0.002, U-test of Mann and Whitney, 2-tailed.

Legal Aspects of the LD_{50}. For the two important goals of acute toxicity testing, the assessment of the hazardous properties of chemicals and the classification for labeling purposes, animal experiments are necessary. However, the numerical value of the LD_{50} obtained in these tests is of little importance for the former, but has traditionally been a decisive factor for the latter. Although it is acknowledged that the LD_{50} is not a biological constant and that it can be influenced by all kinds of experimental manipulations, it has obvious legal advantages: once a LD_{50} figure has been established, classification of the substance is almost automatic. Regulatory agencies fear that if a more scientific, but also more ambiguous general assessment of a chemical's hazard were used as classification criterion, the legal basis would become uncertain, and the debate with industry over classification and reclassification of chemicals and consumer products would lead to a never-ending struggle.

In this context, it should be pointed out that classification guidelines, although they all use LD_{50} values as criteria, differ with regard to the cut-off points (Table 3). This clearly demonstrates that classification and labeling requirements are based on regulatory and legal decisions, rather than on a sound scientific assessment of the risks to public health.

SCIENTIFIC CHALLENGES

It is reasonable to suggest that the highest scientific priorities should be given to those matters that were identified as the major problem areas in the preceding section of this paper. First, traditional acute toxicity testing which describes a dose-effect relationship only for the lethal effect must be changed to include other end-points of toxicity related to morbidity. A proposal for such a "toxicological screening" in which dose-effect relationships are established for a large number of adverse effects, and

TABLE 3
Criteria for Classification of Toxic Chemicals, LD$_{50}$ Oral

United Nations Recommendation	EEC Norway Sweden	US Consumer Protection Label	Swiss Toxic Substance Label	Japan. Toxic and Delet. Subst. Label
Group I 5 mg/kg	very toxic 25 mg/kg	highly toxic 50 mg/kg	Category I 5 mg/kg	Toxic Subst. 30 mg/kg
Group II 5-50 mg/kg			Category II 5-50 mg/kg	
Group III 50-500 mg/kg (solids)	toxic 25/200 mg/kg		Category III 50-500 mg/kg	Deleterious 30-300 mg/kg
500-2000 mg/kg (liquids)	harmful 200-2000 mg/kg		Category IV 500-2000 mg/kg (products) 500-5000 (substances)	
			Category V 2000 mg/kg (products) 5000-15000 mg/kg (substances)	

Source: OECD, internal report, 1983.

which uses small numbers of animals, has recently been published (Zbinden et al., 1984).

Another important aspect is the development of novel biostatistical approaches which exploit the information gained in a limited number of animals to a maximal extent. An interesting suggestion was made by Racine et al. (1986). It shows how reliable estimates of LD$_{50}$ values can be made from limited animal data using Bayesian statistics. In a recent paper, Finney (1985) has highlighted the statistical possibilities and pitfalls of various test procedures using small numbers of animals for the determination of the LD$_{50}$.

The third, and probably most demanding scientific problem, is the redefinition of classification concepts of hazardous chemicals. It is not contested that the danger from acute exposure to large doses is only one of many factors contributing to the overall hazard of a given substance. It follows that the consequences of acute poisoning, as they are measured in acute toxicity tests, should not be the only criterion for the classification of a chemical in official lists of poisonous substances.

However, no generally acknowledged rules exist with regard to other important properties, listed in Table 4. The development of concepts for their incorporation into

TABLE 4
Biological Properties of Chemical Compounds that
Should Be Considered in Hazard Assessment

Toxic effects of single large doses (acute toxicity, LD_{50})

Cumulative toxicity on repeated administration

Absorption from gastrointestinal and respiratory tract, through skin and mucous membranes

Elimination, half-life and accumulation in deep compartments

Penetration through biological barriers (e.g., blood-brain barrier, placental transfer)

Excretion in milk

Teratogenic potential

Mutagenic potential

Carcinogenic potential

Sensitizing properties

Local irritant properties

classification guidelines is a major task that will require a major effort by the scientific community.

ETHICAL CONSIDERATIONS

An important concern underlying the efforts to redesign acute toxicity tests is the reduction of the number of laboratory animals. One approach is the use of the limit test, a procedure that is already accepted by the majority of regulatory agencies. In this test, which is used for compounds of low toxicity, small numbers of rodents, not more than 5, are given a single dose, usually 5000 mg/kg by the oral or 2000 mg/kg by the parenteral route. If none of the animals dies, the substance is considered nontoxic and no further acute toxicity tests are done.

With the limit test, the large numbers of animals that were needlessly killed in earlier times can be saved. However, a few questions still remain to be discussed. For example, most classification guidelines take as the upper limit of an oral dose considered to be harmful a LD_{50} figure of 2000 mg/kg (Table 3). Thus, it seems quite unreasonable to select a LD_0 of 5000 mg/kg as the dose used in the limit test. A lowering of this dose to 2000 mg/kg is, therefore, recommended. Another option not yet generally accepted is the grading of nonlethal signs of toxicity and their consideration in the classification procedure.

Another possibility for reduction of animals is the use of one sex only in most acute toxicity tests. Although quantitative differences in LD_{50} values between male and female rodents are the rule rather than the exception, the signs of intoxication and the target organs of toxicity are usually identical. Thus, no substantial information is lost if only one sex is included in the tests. However, in order to detect exceptional sex differences, it is recommended that acute toxicity studies be performed with one sex, and that a few (not more than 5) subjects of the other sex be treated with one dose selected to be close to the maximally tolerated level.

Although the measures described up to this point would reduce the number of animals used in acute toxicity studies, they would not alleviate the suffering of those subjects that are included in the test procedures. It is in the nature of the LD_{50} test that part of the animals die in the course of the study. Whether this happens early from convulsions or asphyxia, or late as a consequence of gastrointestinal bleeding or organ damage, the degree of suffering is enormous. For this reason, LD_{50} tests with doses causing mortality have been abandoned long ago with large animals, such as dogs and primates. Instead, single dose testing, which starts with low doses, followed by higher doses until the minimal toxic or maximally tolerated dose in reached, is performed. Although a lethal dose is rarely given, substantial information about acute toxicity of the test compounds is obtained and the degree of suffering is minimal. It is not understandable why a similar sequential procedure should not be declared mandatory for àcute toxicity tests with rodents.

Ethical considerations also dictate that animals included in acute toxicity tests must be killed when they show evident signs of pain and distress. In practice one sometimes encounters a certain reluctance to abide by this rule, because the numerical value of the LD_{50} is moved downward by the termination of animals that would have survived the procedure. In certain cases, this can alter the classification and labeling of a chemical and greatly reduce its commercial potential. For this reason, it is important that signs of toxicity be weighed in the assessment of acute toxicity, and that the mortality figures be corrected in those cases where animals were killed for humane reasons. The proposal of the British Toxicology Society (1984) represents a first attempt to deal with this problem.

Finally, toxicologists should be obliged to perform acute toxicity tests in such a way that excessive pain and distress of the animals are avoided. This is particularly important with compounds that have potent local irritant or even caustic effects. If it is not possible to reduce such properties by adjustment of the pH or by the use of a special vehicle, the upper dose permitted in acute toxicity experiments must be determined by the local tolerance and not by systemic toxicity or mortality.

ARE ALTERNATIVE METHODS POSSIBLE?

In recent years much research has been concerned with the replacement of experiments using live animals by *in vitro* tests. It must be asked whether model systems using bacteria, cell cultures or tissues could contribute to the assessment of acute toxicity of chemical substances. This idea is based on the assumption that adverse effects on structure and function of single cells could predict toxicity in the whole animal.

Unfortunately, even in the discussion of alternative methods, acute toxicity is still often identified with determination of the LD_{50}. And as an alternative to conventional acute toxicity tests, it is hoped that a direct correlation could be established between the cytotoxic concentration of a chemical in some *in vitro* systems and the numerical value of its LD_{50} in rodents. Experience has shown that this is possible only for selected groups of substances (Ekwall, 1983). Since death is often due to interaction with specific receptors or regulatory systems functioning in the whole animal only, it is logical that no simple correlation exists between single cell toxicity *in vitro* and systemic toxicity. Moreover, the pharmacokinetic and metabolic fate of the test substances often determines toxicity in the whole organism, but these factors cannot be stimulated satisfactorily in the *in vitro* systems. This is particularly relevant if one considers the great differences in acute toxicity related to the routes of exposure.

As in many other areas of biomedical research, *in vitro* test systems should not be developed with the aim of replacing an established test which uses live animals. Instead, they should be regarded as a research approach of a different dimension. The information they provide is often very valuable, but it concerns events at the cellular and subcellular level. As such it is unique and can usually not be gained in whole animal systems.

Experimental models that assess important biological characteristics such as membrane permeability, stability, and surface charges, active and passive transport of ions and other compounds through the membrane, cellular respiration and energy metabolism, and integrity of the cytoskeleton can provide important data on the basic toxicological characteristics of chemical substances. The investigations can be extended to more specific effects assessed in specialized cells, e.g., axon flow in neurons, contraction in myocytes and synthesis of specific proteins in hepatocytes. Knowledge gained in such models can certainly be used as screening parameters to characterize chemical substances and to compare chemically related compounds. In many cases it might also be possible to establish a ranking order of toxicity, permitting the selection of the least toxic compound in a series of chemically related agents. Moreover such tests may provide guidance for the study of toxic effects *in vivo*. If applied systematically, it is hoped that well-designed *in vitro* test batteries will result in a drastic reduction of the need for whole-animal acute toxicity testing.

REFERENCES

A.B.P.I. (1977). Report on the LD_{50}-Test for the Advisory Committee on the Administration of the Cruelty to Animals Act, 1876. Unpublished document issued by the Association of the British Pharmaceutical Industry, London.
BRIMBLECOMBE, R.W. and LESLIE, G.B. (1984). Cimetidine. In: *Safety Testing of New*

Drugs, Laboratory Predictions and Clinical Performance (D.R. Laurence, A.E.M. McLean, and M. Weatherall, eds), pp. 65–91. Academic Press, London.

BRITISH TOXICOLOGY SOCIETY. (1984). A new approach to the classification of substances and preparations on the basis of their acute toxicity. Human Toxicol. **3**:85–92.

BROWNLEE, K.A., HODGES, J.L., Jr. and ROSENBLATT, M. (1953). The up-and-down method with small samples. J. Amer. Statist. Assoc. **48**:262–277.

BRUCE, R.D. (1985). The up-and-down procedure for acute toxicity testing. Fund. Appl. Toxicol. **5**:151–157.

DAYAN, A., CLARK, B., JACKSON, M., MORGAN, H. and CHARLESWORTH, F.A. (1984). Role of the LD_{50} test in the pharmaceutical industry. Lancet 8376:555–556.

DEICHMANN, W.B. and LE BLANC, T.J. (1943). Determination of the approximate lethal dose with about six animals. J. Ind. Hyg. Toxicol. **25**:415–417.

DEICHMANN, W.B. and MERGARD, E.G. (1948). Comparative evaluation of methods employed to express the degree of toxicity of a compound. J. Ind. Hyg. Toxicol. **30**:373–378.

DIXON, W.J. and MOOD, A.M. (1948). A method for obtaining and analyzing sensitivity data. J. Amer. Stat. Assoc. **43**:109–126.

ECETOC. (1985). Acute toxicity tests, LD_{50} (LC_{50}) determinations and alternatives. European Chemical Industry Ecology & Toxicology Centre, Monograph No. 4, Brussels, Belgium.

EKWALL, B. (1983). Correlation between cytotoxicity and LD_{50}-values. Pharmacologia and Toxicologia, **52**:Suppl. II, 80–99.

FINNEY, D.J. (1985). The median lethal dose and its estimation. Arch. Toxicol. **56**:215–218.

LE BEAU, J.E. (1983). The role of the LD_{50} determination in drug safety evaluation. Regulatory Toxicol. Pharmacol. **3**:71–74.

LORKE, D. (1983). A new approach to practical acute toxicity testing. Arch. Toxicol. **54**:275–287.

MAUGH, T.H. (1983). How many chemicals are there? Science **220**:293.

MUELLER, H. and KLEY, H.P. (1982). Retrospective study on the reliability of an "approximate LD_{50}" determined with a small number of animals. Arch. Toxicol. **51**:189–196.

RACINE, A., GRIEVE, A.P., FLUEHLER, H. and SMITH, A.F.M. (1986). Bayesian methods in practice: Experiences in the pharmaceutical industry. J. Royal Statist. Soc.- Applied Statist. (in press).

SCHUETZ, E. and FUCHS, H. (1982). A new approach to minimizing the number of animals used in acute toxicity testing and optimizing the information of test results. Arch. Toxicol. **51**:197–220.

SPERLING, F. (1976). Nonlethal parameters as indices of toxicity: Inadequacy of the acute LD_{50}. In: *New Concepts of Safety Evaluation* (M. Mehlman, R.E. Shapiro and H. Blumenthal, eds.), pp. 177–191. John Wiley and Sons, New York.

TATTERSALL, M.L. (1982). Statistics and the LD_{50} study. Arch. Toxicol. Suppl. **5**:267–270.

THOMPSON, W.R. (1947). Use of moving averages and interpolation to estimate median-effective dose. I. Fundamental formulas, estimation of error and relation to other methods. Bacteriol. Rev. **11**:115–145.

TREVAN, J.W. (1927). The error of determination of toxicity. Proc. Roy. Soc. **101B**:483–514.

WEIL, C.S. (1952). Tables for convenient calculation of median-effective dose (LD_{50} or ED_{50}) and instructions in their use. Biometrics **8**:249–263.

ZBINDEN, G. (1973). Acute toxicity. *Progress in Toxicology, Special Topics*, Vol. 1, pp. 23–27. Springer Verlag, Berlin.

ZBINDEN, G. (1983). Acute toxicity testing, purpose. In: *Alternative Approaches to Acute Toxicology* (A.M. Goldberg, ed.), pp. 2–22. Mary Ann Liebert Inc., New York.

ZBINDEN, G. and FLURY-ROVERSI, M. (1981). Significance of the LD_{50}-test for the toxicological evaluation of chemical substances. Arch. Toxicol. **47**:77–99.

ZBINDEN, G., ELSNER, J. and BOELSTERLI, U.A. (1984). Toxicological screening. Regulatory Toxicol. Pharmacol. **4**:275–286.

METHODOLOGIES FOR INTERPRETATION OF SHORT-TERM TEST RESULTS WHICH MAY ALLOW REDUCTION IN THE USE OF ANIMALS IN CARCINOGENICITY TESTING

FANNY K. ENNEVER AND HERBERT S. ROSENKRANZ

Department of Environmental Health Sciences
Case Western Reserve University School of Medicine
Cleveland, Ohio

Assessment of the risk to humans posed by chemical substances currently relies primarily on experimental exposure of animals in lifetime feeding studies. Short-term tests for genotoxicity are much less costly and use fewer or no animals, but have not replaced the long-term animal bioassay because their results do not coincide completely. We have developed methodologies for interpretation of short-term tests which improve the usefulness of their results, and may allow them to replace the long-term animal bioassay in some circumstances.

INTRODUCTION

Japanese investigators demonstrated early in this century that chemical substances which caused cancer in humans also caused cancer in animals (Yamagiwa and Itchikawa, 1918). Currently, nearly all substances known to be carcinogenic to humans have also been found to be carcinogenic to animals (Vainio et al., 1985; Wilbourn et al., 1986), supporting the role of the long-term animal carcinogenesis bioassay in determining human risk. However, animal bioassays are expensive (approximately $1 million per chemical), involve the sacrifice of up to 1000 rodents, and give results which are often difficult to interpret (Clayson, 1987).

A number of short-term tests have been developed which measure mutation, chromosomal damage, or cell transformation, and they initially showed great promise as surrogates for carcinogenicity testing (Ames et al., 1975). However, more recent results, particularly from the National Toxicology Program (NTP), have indicated that the situation is more complicated (Zeiger, 1987; Tennant et al., 1987), and that short-term test results do not correspond exactly with the long-term animal bioassay.

---

1. Address correspondence to: Fanny K. Ennever, Ph.D., Department of Environmental Health Sciences, Case Western Reserve University School of Medicine, Cleveland, Ohio 44106.

2. Key words: carcinogenicity prediction; computer methods; risk identification; short-term tests.

3. Abbreviations: CA, carcinogen; CPBS, Carcinogenicity Prediction and Battery Selection; IARC, International Agency for Research on Cancer; MC, moderate carcinogen; NC, non-carcinogen; NTP, National Toxicology Program; SC, strong carcinogen; TD_{50}, tumorigenic dose; WC, weak carcinogen.

The tests can still be very useful, however, particularly since the animal bioassay itself may have some flaws (Ennever et al., 1987; Clayson, 1987; Lave et al., 1988), and also since a prediction need not be perfect in order to be informative (Ennever and Rosenkranz, 1986a, 1988b; Lave and Omenn, 1986). We describe in the remainder of this paper some of the new methodologies for data analysis and interpretation which improve the usefulness of short-term tests and may indicate how animal bioassays could be reduced in number or made more effective.

PREDICTION METHODOLOGIES

CPBS. We have recently developed the Carcinogenicity Prediction and Battery Selection (CPBS[tm,a]) methodology for the interpretation of short-term test results (Pet-Edwards et al., 1985a). The method recognizes that all tests may have false negatives (the test is negative for a chemical which is in fact a carcinogen) and false positives (the test is positive for a non-carcinogen). Bayesian analysis is used to compare the likelihood that the test result or results arose in response to a carcinogen (all positives are true positives and all negatives are false negatives) to the likelihood that they arose in response to a non-carcinogen (all negatives are true negatives and all positives are false positives). What is needed for this analysis is knowledge of the performance characteristics of the tests: sensitivity, symbolized α^+, the proportion of true positives, and specificity, symbolized α^-, the proportion of true negatives. Bayes' equation is used in the following form:

$$P(CA|r) = \frac{P(r|CA)P(CA)}{P(r|CA)P(CA) + P(r|NC)P(NC)} \tag{1}$$

where CA indicates carcinogen and NC indicates non-carcinogen, $P(CA|r)$ is the probability of carcinogenicity given the test result or results (r), $P(r|CA)$ is α^+ if r is positive and $1 - \alpha^+$ if r is negative, $P(r|NC)$ is α^- if r is negative and $1 - \alpha^-$ if r is positive, and $P(CA)$ is the prior (before testing) probability of carcinogenicity. [$P(NC)$ is $1 - P(CA)$.] The prior probability influences the predicted probability, to an extent which reflects the added information provided by the test results. The greater the certainty of the prediction [i.e., the closer $P(CA|r)$ is to 1.0 or 0.0], the less dependent it is on the prior probability (Ennever and Rosenkranz, 1986a).

CPBS analysis provides a predicted probability of carcinogenicity; the interpretation of that probability depends upon the circumstances under which the testing was performed (Ennever and Rosenkranz, 1986a). For example, to maximize overall classification accuracy for NTP non-carcinogens (Shelby and Stasiewicz, 1984), using a prior probability of 0.5, probabilities of 0.3 or below were taken to predict non-carcinogenicity, probabilities of 0.7 or above were taken to predict carcinogenicity, and probabilities in between were considered inconclusive, requiring further testing (Ennever and Rosenkranz, 1986b).

In a risk-averse situation, where the goal is to avoid falsely classifying a carcinogen as

---

[a] CPBS[tm] is a trademark of Case Western Reserve University.

non-carcinogenic, the cut-off probability for predicting non-carcinogenicity can be set much lower, to 0.10 or 0.05 (Yander et al., 1987; Ennever and Rosenkranz, 1987b). Such a probability can be achieved in a number of ways. For analytical purposes, we divide tests into four categories: Class I tests, which have high sensitivity and high specificity; Class II tests, which have high sensitivity but low specificity; Class III tests, which have low sensitivity but high specificity; and Class IV tests, which have low sensitivity and low specificity (Pet-Edwards et al., 1985b).

Table 1 gives a number of batteries of tests in which the probability of carcinogenicity is approximately 0.06 when all results in the battery are negative. The relative proportion of time that all negative results are expected to occur in each battery is also given in Table 1; this relative occurrence is calculated as the denominator in equation (1), and is also influenced by the prior probability (Ennever and Rosenkranz, 1986a). As shown in Table 1, Class I tests contribute most to the predictivity of a battery; however, existing Class I tests are expensive or difficult to perform (Rosenkranz et al., 1986). Class II tests also give good predictivity for negative results, because they have few false negatives, but since they also frequently give false positives, negative results occur less often. For example, negatives in three Class II tests give nearly the same probability as negatives in two Class I tests, but occur less than one-fifth as often (Table 1). Class III tests give many false negatives, so that about twice as many Class III tests as Class II are required to give the same predictivity of negative results, but all-negative results occur more than twice as often in the six Class III tests than in the three Class II tests. Using CPBS analysis, a battery can be selected based on the tests available and the purpose of the testing program (Ennever and Rosenkranz, 1986a).

The probability boundary chosen to divide predicted carcinogens from non-carcinogens is directly related to the relative social costs of falsely classifying carcinogens and non-carcinogens (Ennever and Rosenkranz, 1988a). The social cost of falsely calling a non-carcinogen carcinogenic is that associated with the loss of a potentially useful substance, or the cost of controls to minimize human contact. We will use x to symbolize the cost of a false positive. The social cost of falsely calling a carcinogen non-carcinogenic is that associated with the occurrence of cancers among the exposed population. We will use b to symbolize the ratio of the cost of a false negative to the cost of a false positive. These costs will depend upon the anticipated or current use of the chemical in question; reasonable representative values are $1 million for x and 1 or 10 for b (Lave and Omenn, 1986). CPBS analysis indicates that using a probability cut-off of 0.5 corresponds to considering the costs of false positives and false negatives equal (i.e., b = 1), because a cut-off of 0.5 potentially misclassifies equal numbers of carcinogens and non-carcinogens. Using a cut-off of 0.1 corresponds to considering the cost of a false negative as ten times higher than the cost of a false positive (i.e., b = 10), because a cut-off of 0.1 potentially misclassifies 10 non-carcinogens for every 1 carcinogen (Ennever and Rosenkranz, 1988a).

CPBS analysis enhances the usefulness of short-term tests by providing an objective framework for interpretation of results. Using short-term tests as a pre-screen can

TABLE 1
Probabilities of Carcinogenicity Given by All Negative Results
in Selected Test Batteries (Ennever and Rosenkranz, 1986a)

Number of Negative Results	Type of Tests[a]	Probability of Carcinogenicity[b]	Expected Occurrence
2	2 Class I	0.059	34%
3	1 Class I	0.059	17%
	1 Class II		
	1 Class III		
3	3 Class II	0.060	6.7%
4	2 Class II	0.059	8.5%
	2 Class III		
6	6 Class III	0.056	14%

[a]Class I tests: $\alpha^+ = 0.8$ and $\alpha^- = 0.8$; Class II tests: $\alpha^+ = 0.8$ and $\alpha^- = 0.5$; Class III tests: $\alpha^- = 0.5$ and $\alpha^- = 0.8$ (Ennever and Rosenkranz, 1986a).
[b]Probability of carcinogenicity and expected relative occurrence calculated from equation (1) with a prior probability of 0.5 (see text).

restrict the chemicals selected for a long-term animal carcinogenicity bioassay to those with a high probability of either carcinogenicity (in the case of monitoring existing chemicals for high risk) or non-carcinogenicity (in the case of developing new chemicals to have minimum risk).

Cost-Effectiveness of Animal Bioassay. The long-term animal carcinogenicity bioassay is considered the most relevant predictor of human risk. According to the International Agency for Research on Cancer (IARC):

However, in the case of chemicals for which there is *sufficient evidence* of carcinogenicity in experimental animals, it was considered reasonable to recommend that, for practical purposes, such chemicals be regarded as if they presented a carcinogenic risk to humans... The use of the expressions 'for practical purposes' and 'as if they presented a carcinogenic risk' indicates that at the present time a correlation between carcinogenicity in animals and possible human risk cannot be made on a purely scientific basis, but only pragmatically. Such a pragmatic correlation may be useful to regulatory agencies in making decisions related to the primary prevention of cancer. (IARC, 1982)

Considering animal carcinogens to be human carcinogens is the risk-averse course, but may not be prudent if the accuracy of the animal bioassay is too low. It is difficult to determine the accuracy of the bioassay directly (see next section), but we can start by comparing the concordance between carcinogenicity to rats and to mice. This concordance is about 70% in several, somewhat overlapping compilations of rodent carcinogenicity experiments (Gold et al., 1984, 1986; Zeiger, 1987; Tennant et al., 1987). This means that about 30% of mouse carcinogens are not carcinogenic to rats, and about 30% of rat carcinogens are not carcinogenic to mice. Rats and mice are probably more similar to each other than either is to humans (Hart and Fishbein, 1985), and so 70% concordance is probably an upper bound on the accuracy of the animal bioassay in predicting human carcinogenicity.

What are the implications of an accuracy of the animal bioassay of only 70%? The answer depends on the social costs of misclassifying chemicals, and also on the cost of the testing (about $1 million per chemical), and the proportion of human carcinogens among the chemicals tested (Lave et al., 1988). If chemicals are not tested in the animal bioassay, the assumed alternatives are to treat them as non-carcinogens (allowing human exposure) or as carcinogens (restricting or banning human exposure). For a set of chemicals with 10% human carcinogens, Table 2 shows the critical values of x (the social cost of a false positive in millions of dollars) and b (the ratio of the social costs of a false negative and a false positive) for which animal carcinogenicity testing is cost-effective, and the preferred alternative (treating chemicals as carcinogens or non-carcinogens without testing) for values of x less than those shown in the Table. The cost of a false positive, which is essentially the expected profits of a chemical which would be lost by banning it (Lave et al., 1988), must be $2.8 million or greater for testing ever to be cost-effective. The ratio of the costs of false negatives and false positives, which essentially reflects a societal judgment about the value of preventing cancers, must be greater than 3.9 for testing ever to be cost-effective.

The values in Table 2 were generated assuming that the concordance, sensitivity, and specificity of the rodent bioassay were all 70%. Greater accuracy would decrease the critical values of b and x, and hence increase the number of chemicals for which animal testing would be cost-effective. For example, if the animal bioassay were 90% accurate, when b = 9, x would have to be 1.4 or greater, compared to 2.8 with 70% accuracy. (Conversely, if the animal bioassay were only 60% accurate, when b = 9, x would have to be 5.6 or greater.) Thus, even under the most optimistic assumptions, only for chemicals likely to be quite profitable if allowed to be produced will the

TABLE 2
Critical Values of b and x for which Animal Bioassay Testing
is Cost-Effective (Lave et al., 1988)

b	x	Remark
< 3.86	—	Never test, classify chemicals as non-carcinogens
4	>100	Otherwise classify chemicals as non-carcinogens
8	> 3.45	Otherwise classify chemicals as non-carcinogens
9	> 2.78	Otherwise classify chemicals as carcinogens or non-carcinogens
10	> 3.03	Otherwise classify chemicals as carcinogens
15	> 5.56	Otherwise classify chemicals as carcinogens
20	> 33.33	Otherwise classify chemicals as carcinogens

b: Ratio of social cost of a false negative to a false positive; x: cost of a false positive in millions of dollars (see text). These values assume that the animal bioassay is 70% concordant, sensitive, and specific, and that 10% of tested chemicals are human carcinogens (Lave et al., 1988).

animal bioassay be more cost-effective than treating chemicals as carcinogens or non-carcinogens without testing (Lave et al., 1988).

The animal carcinogenicity bioassay is not worthwhile for routine screening in most circumstances, primarily because of its expense. A battery of short-term tests costs much less than an animal bioassay. For example, of twelve batteries containing up to eight tests considered in Rosenkranz and Ennever (1988), the most expensive cost about $100,000, and all but one of the rest cost less than $50,000. With this lower cost, even with a fairly low accuracy, short-term testing can be cost-effective (Lave and Omenn, 1986). Short-term test batteries could provide an alternative for chemicals with values of b and x too low to make animal testing cost-effective.

Accuracy of the Animal Bioassay. The accuracy of the animal bioassay in predicting carcinogenic risk to humans is unlikely to be greater than 70%, as discussed above, because the concordance between carcinogenicity in rats and mice is only 70%. The animal bioassay is quite sensitive to human carcinogens (Vainio et al., 1985; Wilbourn et al., 1986). Its specificity is more difficult to determine, because the limitations of epidemiology make it difficult to identify chemicals which are not carcinogenic to humans. We have tentatively identified 29 chemicals as "probable human non-carcinogens" (Ennever et al., 1987) based on negative epidemiological findings reported by IARC. The proportions of positive results for definitive human carcinogens and negative results for probable human non-carcinogens given by the animal bioassay are shown in Table 3. Using the standard interpretation of two-species bioassays, in which a single positive result is taken as positive, and four negative results are required to give a negative (Clayson and Krewski, 1986), all but one of the 20 probable human non-carcinogens definitely tested were positive in the animal carcinogenicity bioassay. The results from rats alone had a somewhat higher specificity, but still less than 30% (see Table 3). The low specificity found in this investigation may indicate that the animal bioassay is giving many false positives, that is, many rodent carcinogens may not pose a carcinogenic risk to humans (Ennever et al., 1987). As discussed in the previous section, a false positive has an associated societal cost in the abandonment of a potentially useful chemical. Thus, treating all animal carcinogens as human carcinogens may be an overly risk-averse strategy.

Most of the short-term tests with data for human carcinogens and probable non-carcinogens also had a very low specificity, but three tests, listed in Table 3, seemed to be both sensitive and specific for human carcinogenicity. One of these tests, mutagenicity in *Salmonella typhimurium* (the "Ames test"), is currently the most widely used

TABLE 3

Performance of Animal Bioassay and Selected Short-term Tests in Distinguishing Human Carcinogens from Probable Non-Carcinogens (Ennever et al., 1987)

Test	Positive Results for Carcinogens	Negative Results for Probable Non-Carcinogens
Rat carcinogenicity	5/6	6/19
Mouse carcinogenicity	10/11	2/17
Overall bioassay	10/10	1/19
<u>Salmonella typhimurium</u> mutation	10/12	10/17
<u>Drosophila melanogaster</u> recessive lethals	8/10	7/8
Syrian hamster embryo transformation	5/5	2/3

mutagenicity assay. Although more investigation is needed to follow up on these preliminary findings, it seems that at least some short-term tests may correspond more closely than the animal bioassay to human risk.

Carcinogenic Potency. The regulation of human exposure to carcinogens relies on risk assessment; that is, the calculation of levels of exposure resulting in acceptable risk, typically 10^{-6} (Wilson and Crouch, 1987). Ideally, information is available on the mechanism of action, absorption, metabolism and excretion of the chemical in several species, including humans (Clayson, 1987). However, if such detailed studies are lacking, a risk assessment can still be made simply on the basis of measured carcinogenic potency in animals, although in this case the extrapolation to human risk involves a number of assumptions. When no animal bioassay has been performed, then the carcinogenic potency is not available. If short-term tests could be used to predict carcinogenic potency, then at least a crude risk assessment could perhaps be done without animal bioassays.

Past attempts to predict carcinogenic potency from short-term tests have tried to correlate potency in the short-term test with carcinogenic potency, and have been unsuccessful except in restricted classes of chemicals (Meselson and Russell, 1977; Bartsch et al., 1983; Lewtas, 1986). We have found a correlation between qualitative results in short-term tests (i.e., positive or negative) and carcinogenic potency (Ennever and Rosenkranz, 1987a). Carcinogenic potency results were taken from Gold and co-workers, in which potency was expressed as TD_{50}, the "tumorigenic dose," which reduces by 50% the chance of remaining tumorless (Peto et al., 1984). Carcinogens were divided into three classes of potency: strong carcinogens (SC), with a TD_{50} less than 1 mg/kg/day; moderate carcinogens (MC), with a TD_{50} between 1 and 100 mg/kg/day; and weak carcinogens (WC), with a TD_{50} greater than 100 mg/kg/day. The sensitivities of sixteen short-term tests to the three classes of carcinogens were calculated, and the tests divided into two categories: "under-responsive," with low sensitivity to weak and moderate carcinogens but high sensitivity to strong carcinogens and also high specificity, and "over-responsive," with high sensitivity to carcinogens of all strengths, but low specificity (Ennever and Rosenkranz, 1987a).

These observed patterns of test responses to carcinogenic potency can be used for prediction, by extending Bayes' theorem [equation (1)] to four categories of chemicals. Complete equations are given in Ennever and Rosenkranz (1987a); as an example, given a positive result for a chemical in a particular test, the probability that it is a strong carcinogen is given by:

$$P(SC|+) = \frac{P(+|SC)P(SC)}{P(+|SC)P(SC) + P(+|MC)P(MC) + P(+|WC)P(WC) + P(+|NC)P(NC)} \tag{2}$$

The publication by Gold and co-workers of a supplement to their original set of chemicals (Gold et al., 1986) provided us the opportunity to test the predictivity of short-term tests for carcinogenic potency on a data base independent of that used to derive the sensitivities. Table 4 lists 17 chemicals with new data in Gold et al. (1986) which also had at least two short-term test results. Short-term test results for the 17 chemicals were taken from published reports of the GeneTox and NTP programs (Palajda and Rosenkranz, 1985; Ennever and Rosenkranz, 1987a). The potency is predicted from the sensitivities of the tests to the three categories of carcinogens found in the original investigation, which used data from the first publication of Gold and co-workers (Ennever and Rosenkranz, 1987a).

In Table 4, any increase over the prior probability of 0.25 is considered a positive prediction. Some of the predictions are quite definitive [for example, for caprolactam, $P(NC|r) = 0.80$, and $P(WC|r) = 0.09$, $P(MC|r) = 0.10$, and $P(SC|r) = 0.01$, and for nitrosoethylurethan, $P(SC|r) = 0.68$, and $P(NC|r) = 0.03$, $P(WC|r) = 0.04$, and $P(MC|r) = 0.25$], but others are much less so [for example, for zearalenone, $P(NC|r) = 0.30$, $P(WC|r) = 0.27$, and $P(MC|r) = 0.30$, and $P(SC|r) = 0.14$, and for benzoin, $P(NC|r) = 0.35$, $P(MC|r) = 0.26$, and $P(SC|r) = 0.30$, and $P(WC|r) = 0.08$]. For 12 out of the 17 chemicals, the actual potency was in a category predicted. Only one non-carcinogen, allyl isothiocyanate, was predicted to be carcinogenic, and only one carcinogen, ethanol, was predicted to be non-carcinogenic. This is quite a good performance, particularly since the short-term test batteries were simply results available from the published literature, not selected for potency predictivity.

The qualitative short-term test results predict potency semi-quantitatively, that is, into one of three potency categories. Three categories were used in the original investigation to provide a sufficient number of chemicals in each class to estimate sensitivity of the tests (Ennever and Rosenkranz, 1987a), but it is possible that if more data were available, more potency categories could be used. However, even the three categories, each encompassing two orders of magnitude, provide useful information, particularly considering that the animal bioassay results often give potency estimates which differ by a factor of 100 for the same chemical (Gaylor and Chen, 1986; Ames et al., 1987), and that other assumptions required for risk assessment may not be certain to more than a factor of 100 (Ennever et al., 1988). Thus, short-term test results may be able to provide sufficient information on carcinogenic potency to reduce the need for animal bioassays.

CONCLUSIONS

Both short-term tests and animal bioassays are tools for risk identification, which is only a first step in risk assessment. Full assessment of the relevance of an identified risk should take into account dose, absorption, metabolism, distribution, reaction with DNA, repair of DNA, and tumor expression (Clayson, 1987). Animal models will always be required for such investigations.

What our methodologies for short-term test interpretation may allow is predicting

TABLE 4
Actual and Predicted Potency of 17 New Chemicals

Chemical	Test Results	Potency Predicted	Actual
Actual potency is in category predicted:			
Caffeine	Sty− EcW− plA+ SCE+ Cvt+ DRL+ SHE− VT7−	**NC**	NC
Caprolactam	Sty− SCE− Cvt−	**NC**	NC
11−Aminoundecanoic acid	Sty− DRL−	NC/**WC**	WC
Cinnamyl anthranilate	Sty− DRL−	NC/**WC**	WC
Phenol	Sty− DRL−	NC/**WC**	WC
Zearalenone	Sty− Bsr+	NC/**MC**/WC	MC
Benzidine dihydrochloride	Sty+ DRL− VT7+	**MC**/NC	MC
Benzoin	Sty+ SCE+ Cvt−	**NC**/SC/MC	NC
Ethylene oxide	Sty+ DRL+ Mnt+	SC/**MC**	MC
3−Methoxy−4−aminoazobenzene	Sty+ plA+ HMA+ SHE+	SC/**MC**	MC
1,2−Propylene oxide	DRL+ VT7+	SC/**MC**	MC
Nitrosoethylurethan	Sty+ plA+ DRL+	**SC**	SC
Actual potency is different from predicted			
Ethyl alcohol	Sty− SCE− Cvt− Mnt− SHE− VTR−	NC	WC
Acetaldehyde methylformylhydrazone	EcW− HMA−	NC/WC	MC
Tin (II) chloride	Sty− EcW− Bsr−	NC/WC	MC
4−(5−Nitro−2−furyl)thiazole	Sty+ Bsr+ SHE−	NC/SC	MC
Allyl isothiocyanate	Sty+ DRL+	SC	NC

Test abbreviations: Sty, *Salmonella typhimurium* mutation assay; EcW, *E. coli* WP2 reverse mutation assay; plA, *E. coli* DNA repair using polA$^+$ and polA$^-$ strains; SCE, sister chromatid exchanges; Cvt, chromosomal aberrations *in vitro*; DRL, *Drosophila melanogaster* recessive lethals; SHE, Syrian hamster embryo transformation; VT7, chemical enhancement of SA7 adenovirus transformation; Bsr, *Bacillus subtilis* repair using rec$^+$ and rec$^-$; Mnt, the micronucleus test; HMA, the host mediated assay.

Classes of carcinogenic potency: strong carcinogens (SC), with a TD$_{50}$ ("tumorigenic dose") less than 1 mg/kg/day; moderate carcinogens (MC), with a TD$_{50}$ between 1 and 100 mg/kg/day; weak carcinogens (WC), with a TD$_{50}$ greater than 100 mg/kg/day, and non-carcinogens (NC), with no carcinogenic effect in male and female rats and mice (see text). Actual potency taken from Gold et al. (1986), potency predicted from sensitivities to SC, MC, and WC calculated from Gold et al. (1984), counting any increase over the prior probability of 0.25 as a positive prediction (Ennever and Rosenkranz, 1987a).

carcinogenicity without lifetime exposure of up to 1000 rodents per chemical. The development of these methodologies, however, required comparing results from short-term tests to results from animal bioassays, and additional data from animal experiments will always be necessary to refine the predictive ability of short-term tests. Also, animal models have an essential role in elucidating mechanisms of carcinogenesis. The routine requirement of the animal bioassay to screen chemicals for carcinogenicity is what could be minimized by further improvement and acceptance of our CPBS methodologies.

ACKNOWLEDGEMENTS

Supported by the Mary Ann Swetland Program in Medicine and Human Behavior, the Dana Foundation, the National Institute of Environmental Health Sciences and the U.S. Environmental Protection Agency.

REFERENCES

AMES, B.N., McCANN, J. and YAMASAKI, E. (1975). Methods for detecting carcinogens and mutagens with the *Salmonella*/mammalian-microsome mutagenicity test. Mutation Res. **31**:347–364.

AMES, B.N., MAGAW, R. and GOLD, L.S. (1987). Ranking possible carcinogenic hazards. Science **236**:271–280.

CLAYSON, D.B. (1987). The need for biological risk assessment in reaching decisions about carcinogens. Mutation Res. **185**:243–269.

CLAYSON, D.B. and KREWSKI, D. (1986). The concept of negativity in experimental carcinogenesis. Mutation Res. **167**:233–240.

ENNEVER, F.K. and ROSENKRANZ, H.S. (1986a). Evaluating batteries of short-term genotoxicity tests. Mutagenesis **1**:293–298.

ENNEVER, F.K. and ROSENKRANZ, H.S. (1986b). Short-term test results for NTP non-carcinogens: An alternate, more predictive battery. Environ. Mutagen. **8**:849–865.

ENNEVER, F.K. and ROSENKRANZ, H.S. (1987a). Prediction of carcinogenic potency by short-term genotoxicity tests. Mutagenesis **2**:39–44.

ENNEVER, F.K. and ROSENKRANZ, H.S. (1987b). Selection of batteries in an industrial setting (Reply to letter of Yander et al.). Environ. Mutagen. **9**:359–361.

ENNEVER, F.K. and ROSENKRANZ, H.S. (1988a). Influence of the proportion of carcinogens on the cost effectiveness of short-term tests. Mutation Res. **197**:1–13.

ENNEVER, F.K. and ROSENKRANZ, H.S. (1988b). New methodologies to predict rodent carcinogenicity from genotoxicity assays: Application to recent National Toxicology Program short-term test data. Environ. Molec. Mutagen., submitted.

ENNEVER, F.K., NOONAN, T.J. and ROSENKRANZ, H.S. (1987). The predictivity of animal bioassays and short-term genotoxicity tests for carcinogenicity and non-carcinogenicity to humans. Mutagenesis **2**:73–78.

ENNEVER, F.K., PURVIS, S.F. AND ROSENKRANZ, H.S. (1988). The potential for detecting human cancers resulting from TCDD exposure. Toxicol. Appl. Pharmacol., submitted.

GAYLOR, D.W. and CHEN, J.J. (1986). Relative potency of chemical carcinogens in rodents. Risk Anal. **6**:283–290.

GOLD, L.S., SAWYER, C.B., MAGAW, R., BACKMAN, G.M., DE VECIANA, M., LEVINSON, R., HOOPER, N.K., HAVENDER, W.R., BERNSTEIN, L., PETO, R., PIKE, M.C. and AMES, B.N. (1984). A carcinogenic potency database of the standardized results of animal bioassays. Environ. Health Perspect. **58**:9–319.

GOLD, L.S., DE VECIANA, M., BACKMAN, G.M., MAGAW, R., LOPIPERNO, P., SMITH, M., BLUMENTHAL, M., LEVINSON, R., BERNSTEIN, L. and AMES, B.N. (1986). Chronological supplement to the Carcinogenic Potency Database: Standardized results of animal bioassays published through December 1982. Environ. Health Perspect. **67**:161–200.

HART, R.W. and FISHBEIN, L. (1985). Interspecies extrapolation of drug and genetic toxicity data. In: *Toxicological Risk Assessment, Volume I. Biological and Statistical Criteria* (Clayson, D.B., Krewski, D., and Munro, I., eds.), pp. 3–40, CRC Press, Boca Raton, FL.

INTERNATIONAL AGENCY FOR RESEARCH ON CANCER (1982). IARC Monographs on the Evaluation of the Carcinogenic Risks of Chemicals to Humans, Supplement 4, Chemicals, Industrial Processes and Industries Associated with Cancer in Humans (IARC Monographs, Volumes 1 to 29), 292 pp., Lyon.

LAVE, L.B. and OMENN, G.S. (1986). Cost-effectiveness of short-term tests for carcinogenicity. Nature **324**:29–34.

LAVE, L.B., ENNEVER, F.K., ROSENKRANZ, H.S. and OMENN, G.S. (1988). On the usefulness of the lifetime rodent bioassay for identifying cancer-causing chemicals. Nature, submitted.

LEWTAS, J. (1986). Comparative potency method for cancer risk assessment: Application to the quantitative assessment of the contribution of combustion emissions to lung cancer risk. In: *Genetic Toxicology of Environmental Chemicals, Part B: Genetic Effects and Applied Mutagenesis* (Ramel, C., Lambert, B., and Magnusson, J., eds.), pp. 529–535, Alan R. Liss, Inc., New York.

MESELSON, M. and RUSSELL, K. (1977). Comparison of carcinogenic and mutagenic potency. In: *Origins of Human Cancer, Book C. Human Risk Assessment* (Hiatt, H.H., Watson, J.D., and Winstein, J.A., eds.), pp. 1473–1481, Cold Spring Harbor Laboratory, Cold Spring Harbor, N.Y.

PALAJDA, M. and ROSENKRANZ, H.S. (1985). Assembly and preliminary analysis of a genotoxicity data base for predicting carcinogens. Mutation Res. **153**:79–134.

PET-EDWARDS, J., ROSENKRANZ, H.S., CHANKONG, V. and HAIMES, Y.Y. (1985). Cluster analysis in predicting the carcinogenicity of chemicals using short-term assays. Mutation Res. **153**:167–185.

PET-EDWARDS, J., CHANKONG, V., ROSENKRANZ, H.S. and HAIMES, Y.Y. (1985). Application of the carcinogenicity prediction and battery selection (CPBS) method to the GeneTox data base. Mutation Res. **153**:187–200.

PETO, R., PIKE, M.C., BERNSTEIN, L., GOLD, L.S. and AMES, B.N. (1984). The TD_{50}: A proposed general convention for the numerical description of the carcinogenic potency of chemicals in chronic-exposure animal experiments. Environ. Health Perspect. **58**:1–8.

ROSENKRANZ, H.S. and ENNEVER, F.K. (1988). New approaches to battery selection and interpretation. In: *New Trends in Genetic Risk Assessment* (Jolles, G. and Cordier, A., eds.), Academic Press Inc., London, in press.

ROSENKRANZ, H.S., ENNEVER, F.K., CHANKONG, V., PET-EDWARDS, J. and HAIMES, Y.Y. (1986). An objective approach to the development of short-term tests predictive of carcinogenicity. Cell Biol. Toxicol. **2**:425–440.

SHELBY, M.D. and STASIEWICZ, S. (1984). Chemicals showing no evidence of carcinogenicity in long-term, two-species rodent studies: The need for short-term test data. Environ. Mutagen. **6**:871–878.

TENNANT, R.W., MARGOLIN, B.H., SHELBY, M.D., ZEIGER, E., HASEMAN, J.K., SPALDING, J., CASPARY, W., RESNICK, M., STASIEWICZ, S., ANDERSON, B. and MINOR, R. (1987). Prediction of chemical carcinogenicity in rodents from in vitro genetic toxicity assays. Science **236**:933–941.

VAINIO, H., HEMMINKI, K. and WILBOURN, J. (1985). Data on the carcinogenicity of chemicals in the IARC Monographs programme. Carcinogenesis **6**:1653–1655.

WILBOURN, J., HAROUN, L., HASELTINE, E., KALDOR, J., PARTENSKY, C. and VAINIO, H. (1986). Response of experimental animals to human carcinogens: an analysis based upon the IARC Monographs programme. Carcinogenesis **7**:1853–1863.

WILSON, R. and CROUCH, E.A.C. (1987). Risk assessment and comparisons: an introduction. Science **236**:267–270.

YAMAGIWA, K. and ITCHIKAWA, K. (1918). Experimental study of the pathogenesis of carcinoma. J. Cancer Res. **3**:1–21.

YANDER, G., LIN, G.H. and MERMELSTEIN, R. (1987). Selection of batteries in an industrial setting: Letter to the Editor. Environ. Mutagen. **9**:357–358.

ZEIGER, E. (1987). Carcinogenicity of mutagens: Predictive capability of the *Salmonella* mutagenesis assay for rodent carcinogenicity. Cancer. Res. **47**:1287–1296.

Received January 5, 1988
Accepted January 28, 1988

CASE, THE COMPUTER-AUTOMATED STRUCTURE EVALUATION SYSTEM, AS AN ALTERNATIVE TO EXTENSIVE ANIMAL TESTING

HERBERT S. ROSENKRANZ AND GILLES KLOPMAN

**Departments of Environmental Health Sciences and Chemistry
Case Western Reserve University
Cleveland, Ohio**

CASE, an artificial intelligence system with demonstrated ability to predict biological activity based on structural considerations, correctly predicts animal carcinogenicity. It can, therefore, play a pivotal role in classifying chemicals as carcinogens and prioritizing them for further testing. Additionally, CASE shows promise in the design of pharmacologically active agents by reducing the number of drugs that need to be synthesized and tested. For both of these applications, CASE provides a mechanism to conserve animal and other testing resources.

INTRODUCTION

If we believe that the pharmacological and toxicological properties of a chemical are dependent upon thermodynamic and kinetic principles, which to a large extent, regulate recognition by specific enzymes, receptors, immunoglobins or other similar structures or a combination of these, then since these interactions obey the laws of physics and chemistry, they should be amenable to analysis on the basis of structure-activity relationships (SAR). The corollary to this is the fact that an understanding of SAR should assist in the prediction of the activity of yet untested molecules and be most economical of available resources by reducing the amount of routine testing required to identify molecules of increasingly crucial relevance. It must be realized that in all studies using SAR, a learning set (i.e., a data base) is needed and that it must be based on actual experimentation using either animals, surrogate test systems, or cell-free enzymic reactions. Moreover, from time to time, in order to verify the continued validity of the model being developed and refined, actual testing will be needed. So it is apparent that SAR studies hold much promise for both pharmacolog-

---

1. Address correspondence to: Dr. Herbert S. Rosenkranz, Department of Environmental Health Sciences, School of Medicine, Case Western Reserve University, Cleveland, OH 44106.
2. Key words: alternative methodology, carcinogen, structure-activity relationships.
3. Abbreviations: CASE, Computer-Automated Structure Evaluation System; SAR, structure-activity relationships.

ical and toxicological sciences. The question that is addressed here concerns the relevance of CASE, the Computer Automated Structure Evaluation system, recently developed by us (Klopman, 1984; Klopman and Rosenkranz, 1984), to problems of pharmacological and toxicological concern. The initial focus is on the application of CASE to the study of mutagens and carcinogens. There have been several recent reviews on the applicability of SAR techniques, including CASE, to mutagens and carcinogens (Frierson et al., 1986; Rosenkranz et al., 1986b).

CASE differs from other SAR techniques in being completely automatic, that is, it selects its own fragment descriptors from the practically infinite number of possible structural assemblies. This is an important feature as other SAR procedures are primarily interactive between the operator and the computer, wherein the operator selects possible descriptors that are part of a fixed panel. Unless the correct descriptors are included, and the appropriate one may very well not be part of the panel, then the correlations obtained are not good. Thus, the ADAPT SAR technique yields a very good prediction for the carcinogenicity of polycyclic aromatic hydrocarbons (PAH's) when the bay region is included among the descriptors (Chou and Jurs, 1979). The bay region, of course, has been identified as being crucial to the carcinogenicity of most PAH's (Jerina et al., 1976). However, if this region or an equally important one is as yet unrecognized, and is, therefore, not included among the SAR descriptors, then the prediction suffers accordingly. As we show below, CASE, when applied to a panel of PAH's, will "discover" the bay region as being one of the important determinants of the carcinogenicity of this class of chemicals. In parallel with the ability to generate the descriptors and select the significant ones, CASE has an additional feature which is superior to the chemist's approach. As chemists, we approach traditional SAR by asking questions that are readily visualized by us, for example, does the candidate molecule have an amino group, a carboxylic acid moiety or a halogen? Yet we know well that enzymes and other biological receptors recognize moieties that are much larger than the groupings that we usually consider. It is one of the strengths of CASE that it can generate substructures that have the larger size that is associated with biological activity. The CASE methodology has been described on a number of occasions. For illustrative purposes we will consider here the use of CASE in predicting the carcinogenicity of two PAH's. The first of these, benzo[a]pyrene (B[a]P), is a widely distributed and studied carcinogen that acts by virtue of the presence of the bay region. The second chemical is benz(e)aceanthrylene (B[e]A), a cyclopenta-fused PAH which is also of environmental concern but which has not yet been studied as widely.

METHODOLOGY

The CASE methodology has been described on a number of occasions (Klopman, 1984; Klopman et al., 1985a,b, 1987; Klopman and Macina, 1985; Klopman and Rosenkranz, 1984; Rosenkranz et al., 1984, 1985). Basically, CASE selects its own descriptors automatically from a learning set composed of active and inactive molecules. The descriptors are easily recognizable single, continuous structural fragments that are embedded in the complete molecule. The descriptors consist of either activating (biophore) or inactivating (biophobe) fragments. Once the training set has been assimilated, CASE can be queried regarding the predicted activity of molecules of unknown activity. Thus, entry of an unknown chemical will result in the generation of all the possible fragments ranging from 3 to 10 atoms accompanied by their hydrogens and these will be compared to the previously identified biophores and biophobes. On the basis of the presence and/or absence of these descriptors, CASE predicts activity or lack thereof. In addition, and independently of the above, CASE also uses the descriptors to perform an *ad hoc* multivariate regression analysis (QSAR) which results in a projected potency (Frierson et al., 1986; Klopman et al., 1987a,b).

The data bases used for determining the structural determinants of the carcinogenicity data consisted of 48 PAH's tested in female Sencar Swiss mice by the initiation-promotion skin carcinogenesis protocol (Mitchell et al., 1986). While B[a]P is included in the data base, neither B[e]A nor any of its cyclopenta-fused analogs are in the learning set (Mitchell et al., 1986).

RESULTS AND DISCUSSION

Carcinogenicity. Based upon the mouse two-stage carcinogenicity data base, CASE identified four major descriptors (biophores) responsible for the carcinogenicity of PAH's (Figure 1). One of these biophores (Figure 1, fragment 6), was identified in both B[a]P and B[e]A (Figures 2 and 3); in fact, it is associated with a 100% probability of carcinogenicity. In view of the fact that the same biophore was identified in the two PAH's, it is not surprising that the predicted carcinogenicity (100%), and potency (see below), are identical. The potency is calculated from the QSAR equation (Figure 1): $17.2645 + 13.1980 = 30.46$. This corresponds to a moderate potency, i.e., the dose required for 50% of the animals to develop tumors is expected to be less than 200 nanomoles (Mitchell et al., 1986).

Further examination of the biophore indicates that, as expected, it corresponds to a structure common to both B[a]P and B[e]A and includes, in each instance, the bay regions (Figure 4). Because B[a]P is present in the data base as a mouse skin carcinogen, it is not surprising that CASE identifies it as a carcinogen. However, neither B[e]A nor any of its structural congeners are present in the learning set, yet CASE identified the biophore which predicts its carcinogenicity for the mouse skin. Additionally, the QSAR feature of CASE predicts that both chemicals will have identical potencies, i.e., requiring approximately 200 nanomoles for 50% of the animals to develop tumors. It is comforting to know that a recent study has indeed demonstrated the mouse skin tumor-initiating activity of B[e]A and moreover it also showed that it was of the same magnitude as that of B[a]P, and similar to the potency

```
QSAR EQUATION :

ACTIVITY =    17.2645 + 13.1980 FRAG (6) + 8.42627 FRAG (1)
                       11.0224 FRAG (2) + 8.93683 FRAG (9)


DESCRIPTORS :

Frag nr.  1  CH =CH -CH =CH -C. =C. -C =          Prob.=  0.018 ACTIVE
Frag nr.  2  C  =C. -CH =CH -CH =CH -C. =C -       Prob.=  0.063 ACTIVE
Frag nr.  6  CH =C. -CH =C. -CH =CH -CH =CH -C. =C. -   Prob.=  0.004 ACTIVE
Frag nr.  9  CH3-C =C. -CH =CH -CH =C. -CH =CH -C. =    Prob.=  0.125 ACTIVE
```

FIGURE 1. Major biophores associated with the carcinogenicity of PAHs in the mouse skin two-stage carcinogenicity assay. The QSAR equation permits the calculation of projected carcinogenicity based upon the presence of specific descriptors. Fragment 6 is present in B[a]P and B[e]A, see Figs. 2-4.

predicted by CASE, i.e., approximately 200 nanomoles for 50% of the animals to develop tumors (Nesnow et al., 1984).

It should be noted that in the instance of the PAH's examined here, CASE, without any prior knowledge, identified the bay region as essential to the carcinogenicity of these chemicals. This then can be seen as validation of the CASE methodology. It also

```
C2CC2DD2C/D2DD2C/D2DC/2DC2C/D2DD2D/    BaP

   FORMULA
   --------
  1 2 3 4  5  6  7  8  9  10 11 12 13 14 1516 17 18 19 20
  --------------------------------------------------------
  C               )
                        )
   =C                            )
    -C                               )
     =CH-CH=C -CH=CH-CH=C -CH=CH-C =CH-C              )
                                       =C -CH=CH-CH=CH

100 % chances of being   ACTIVE due to substructure (Conf.level= 100%) :
        CH =C. -CH =C. -CH =CH -CH =CH -C. =C. -

*** OVERALL, the probability of being a Carcinogen   is 100.0% ***

      ** The activity is predicted to be MODERATE ( 30) **
```

FIGURE 2. CASE prediction of the carcinogenicity of B[a]P for mouse skin. The code in the upper left is the KLN code (Klopman, 1984) which permits entry into the CASE program. CASE has identified a biophore associated with a 100% probability of carcinogenicity. Note that this biophore is identical to Fragment 6 of Fig. 1 (see also Fig. 4). The activity, i.e. 30, is calculated from the QSAR equation (Fig. 1).

```
D2DD2DC2C/D2CC2C/D2DC)2DC2C/D2DD2D/        B(E)A

    FORMULA
    -------
 1  2  3  4   5 6   7   8 9 10 11 12 13 14 1516 17 18 19 20
-----------------------------------------------------------------
 CH                  )
    =CH-CH=CH-C              )
              =C  -CH=C                 )
                 -C           )=CH-C                      )
                  =C  -CH=CH-C        =C  -CH=CH-CH=CH
```

```
100 % chance of being  ACTIVE due to substructure (Conf.level= 100%) :
       CH =C. -CH =C. -CH =CH -CH =CH -C. =C. -

*** OVERALL, the probability of being a carcinogen   is 100.0% ***

    ** The activity is predicted to be MODERATE ( 30) **
```

FIGURE 3. CASE prediction of the carcinogenicity of B[e]A. CASE has identified a biophore associated with a 100% probability of carcinogenicity. Note that this biophore is identical to Fragment 6 of Fig. 1 (see also Fig. 4).

suggests that the CASE predictions are based on sound fundamental principles. With respect to its future use, of course, as CASE is an expert system, it will also require experts to ascertain that the interpretation of the results are in keeping with their biological significance.

CASE has been used to predict carcinogenicity and mutagenicity of many classes of chemicals. In view of some of the limitations in the predictivity of rodent bioassays, such as only a 70% concordance between rats and mice (Tennant et al., 1987), which suggests that predictivity of carcinogenicity in humans cannot be expected to exceed

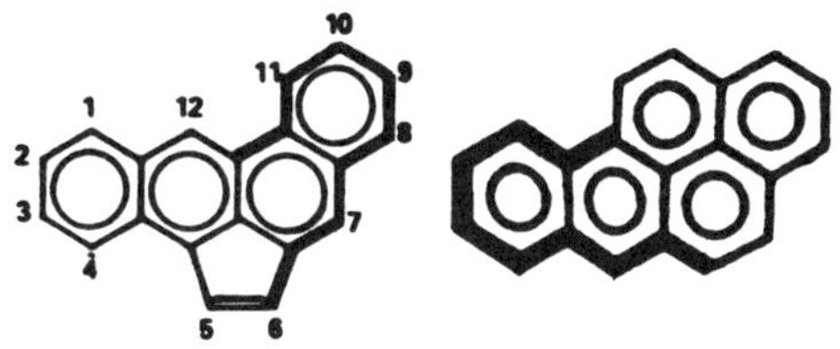

FIGURE 4. The localization of the biophore identified by CASE. B[e]A left and B[a]P to the right. The highlighted structures correspond to the biophore identified by CASE. (Figures 2 and 3, and fragment 6 of Figure 1). The region between atoms 11 and 12 of B[e]A is the bay region.

70%, as well as the high cost of the animal bioassay (approximately $1 million per chemical) (Lave et al., 1988), it would seem that the standard animal carcinogenicity assay is not a reliable predictor of human risk. Moreover, the situation is aggravated further by the realization that the predictivity of the animal bioassay is based upon a chemical selection process in which the prevalence of carcinogens is approximately 70%, yet the expected proportion of carcinogens in the chemical universe is not expected to exceed 10% of chemicals. Thus, it would seem that the usual bioassay is not likely to be either a highly predictive or an economical instrument for assessing human risk (Lave et al., 1988; Ennever and Rosenkranz, 1988). Accordingly, SAR activity concepts, such as the CASE method illustrated herein, present an attractive alternative to prioritize chemicals for further testing prior to extensive animal bioassays.

Other Applications of CASE. Although CASE was originally developed to study the structural basis of mutagenicity and carcinogenicity (Klopman and Rosenkranz, 1984; Klopman et al., 1985a,b, 1986, 1987; Rosenkranz et al., 1985, 1986a,b, 1987a,b), it soon became evident that it could be used to study other biological properties as well, including many pharmacological ones. It is in the arena of the design of pharmacological molecules that CASE shows great promise (Klopman and Kalos, 1986; Klopman and Macina, 1985, 1987; Klopman and Venegas, 1986). Thus a recent study demonstrated the ability of CASE to suggest a structure of an active quinolone antibacterial agent (Klopman et al., 1987b). Although it cannot be expected that CASE will unerringly lead to the design of the ultimate agent in each case, it could, in effect, greatly decrease the total number of pharmacologically active agents that need to be synthesized and tested in animals. Thus, while the usual experience is to start with approximately 400 candidate molecules for further testing and end up with 1 to 3 which have the wanted properties, it is probable that CASE will decrease the number of candidates to between 25 and 40, thus greatly reducing costs as well as being economical of resources. A feature of the CASE program which is unique and is, therefore, of great value, is its ability to compare data bases and thereby design molecules in which therapeutic activities are optimized and toxic side effects minimized.

CONCLUSIONS

The concept of using structural analyses to predict the properties of biological active molecules is not new. Heretofore many of these methods either were completely heuristic or dependent upon the operator's intuition with respect to which chemical moieties were important. Additionally, the final QSAR equations that are derived frequently do not permit mechanistic insight. CASE, on the other hand, is a completely automatic as well as self-learning expert system, which identifies continuous, easily recognizable structures embedded within the larger molecule. These structures can then be studied further with respect to their mechanistic significance such as identification of sites for biotransformation or indications of the size of the receptor site. It has already been demonstrated that the information provided by CASE is extremely useful in understanding the structural basis of biological activity including mutagenicity, carcinogenicity, antimicrobial activity, β-blockers as well as halucinogens. There is every reason to expect that as CASE is applied to additional problems, it will be equally effective. Certainly, at this stage of its development, CASE is a very cost-effective method for reducing the number of molecules that need to be tested in bioassays.

ACKNOWLEDGEMENTS

This investigation was supported by the U.S. Environmental Protection Agency.

REFERENCES

CHOU, J.T. and JURS, P.C. (1979). Computer-assisted structure-activity studies of chemical carcinogens. J. Med. Chem. **22**:792–797.

ENNEVER, F.K. and ROSENKRANZ, H.S. (1988). Methodologies for interpretation of short-term test results which may allow reduction in the use of animals in carcinogenicity testing. Toxicol. Ind. Health, in press.

FRIERSON, M.R., KLOPMAN, G. and ROSENKRANZ, H.S. (1986). Structure-activity relationships among mutagens and carcinogens: A review. Environ. Mutagen. **8**:283–327.

JERINA, D.M., LEHR, R.E., YAGI, H., HERNANDEZ, O., DANSETTE, P.M., WISLOCKI, P.G., WOOD, A.W., CHANG, R.L., LEVIN, W. and CONNEY, A.H. (1976). Mutagenicity of benzo[a]pyrene derivatives and the description of a quantum mechanical model which predicts the ease of carbonium ion formation from diol epoxides. In: F.J. de Serres, J.R. Fouts, J.R. Bend and R.M. Philpot (eds), In Vitro Metabolic Activation in Mutagenesis Testing, pp. 159–178. Amsterdam: Elsevier/North Holland Biomedical Press.

KLOPMAN, G. (1984). Artificial intelligence approach to structure-activity studies. Computer-automated structure evaluation of biological activity of organic molecules. J. Amer. Chem. Soc. **106**:7315–7321.

KLOPMAN, G. and KALOS, A.N. (1986). Quantitative structure-activity relationships of beta-adrenergic agents. Application of the computer-automated structure evaluation (CASE) technique of molecular fragment recognition. J. Theor. Biol. **118**:199–214.

KLOPMAN, G. and MACINA, O.T. (1985). Use of the computer automated structure evaluation program in determining quantitative structure-activity relationships within hallucinogenic phenylalkylamines. J. Theor. Biol. **113**:637–648.

KLOPMAN, G. and MACINA, O.T. (1987). Computer-automated structure evaluation of antileukemic 9-aniloacridines. Molec. Pharmacol. **31**:457–476.

KLOPMAN, G. and ROSENKRANZ, H.S. (1984). Structural requirements for the mutagenicity of environmental nitroarenes. Mutation Res. **126**:227–238.

KLOPMAN, G. and VENEGAS, R.E. (1986). CASE study of *in vitro* inhibition of sparteine monooxygenase. Acta Pharm. Jugosl. **36**:189–209.

KLOPMAN, G., CONTRERAS, R., ROSENKRANZ, H.S. and WATERS, M.D. (1985a). Structure-genotoxic activity relationships of pesticides: Comparison between the results of several short-term assays. Mutation Res. **147**:343–356.

KLOPMAN, G., FRIERSON, M.R. and ROSENKRANZ, H.S. (1985b). Computer analysis of toxicological databases: Mutagenicity of aromatic amines in *Salmonella* tester strains. Environ. Mutagen. 7:625–644.

KLOPMAN, G., KALOS, A., FRIERSON, M. and ROSENKRANZ, H.S. (1986). NPPD (spy dust) is predicted to be a mutagen. Environ. Mutagen. 8:627–630.

KLOPMAN, G., KALOS, A.N. and ROSENKRANZ, H.S. (1987a). An artificial intelligence study of the structure-activity relationships of non-fused ring nitroarenes and related compounds. Molec. Toxicol. 1:61–81.

KLOPMAN, G., MACINA, O.T., LEVINSON, M.E. and ROSENKRANZ, H.S. (1987b). Computer automated structure evaluation of quinolone antibacterials. Antimicrob. Ag. Chemotherap. 31:1831–1840.

LAVE, B., ENNEVER, F.K., ROSENKRANZ, H.S. and OMENN, G.S. (1988). The usefulness of lifetime rodent bioassays for identifying cancer-causing chemicals.

MITCHELL, C.S., KLOPMAN, G. and ROSENKRANZ, H.S. (1986). Computer automated evaluation of mutagenicity and carcinogenicity of selected polycyclic aromatic hydrocarbons. In: Polynuclear Aromatic Hydrocarbons (Ninth International Symposium) (M. Cooke and A.J. Denis, eds), pp. 611–624. Battelle Press, Columbus, Ohio.

NESNOW, S., GOLD, A., SANGAIAH, R., TRIPLETT, L.L. and SLAGA, T.J. (1984). Mouse skin tumor-initiating activity of benze(e)aceanthrylene and benz(1)aceanthrylene in Sencar mice. Cancer Letters 22:263–268.

ROSENKRANZ, H.S. and KLOPMAN, G. (1987a). Computer automated structure evaluation of the carcinogenicity of N-nitrosothiazolidine 4-carboxylic acid. Food Chem. Toxicol. 25:253–256.

ROSENKRANZ, H.S. and KLOPMAN, G. (1987b). Artificial intelligence in the study of structural relationships amongst mutagens and carcinogens. In: Trends in Genetic Toxicology (G. Jolles and A. Cordier, eds), Academic Press, in press.

ROSENKRANZ, H.S., FRIERSON, M.R. and KLOPMAN, G. (1986a). Computer-automated prediction of the mutagenicity of benzidine, 4,4"-diaminoterphenyl, 4-dimethylaminoazobenzene and 4-cyanodimethylaniline: Comparison with the results of the Second UKEMS Collaborative Study. Mutagenesis 1:275–282.

ROSENKRANZ, H.S., FRIERSON, M.R. and KLOPMAN, G. (1986b). Use of structure-activity relationships in predicting carcinogenesis. In: Long-Term and Short-Term Assays for Carcinogens: A Critical Appraisal (R. Montesano et al., eds), IARC Scientific Publication No. 83, pp. 497–577. International Agency for Research on Cancer, Lyon.

ROSENKRANZ, H.S., KLOPMAN, G., CHANKONG, V., PET-EDWARDS, J. and HAIMES, Y.Y. (1984). Prediction of environmental carcinogens: A strategy for the mid-1980's. Environ. Mutagen. 6:231–258.

ROSENKRANZ, H.S., MITCHELL, C.S. and KLOPMAN, G. (1985). Artificial intelligence and Bayesian decision theory in the prediction of chemical carcinogens. Mutation Res. 150:1–11.

TENNANT, R.W., MARGOLIN, B.H., SHELBY, M.D., ZEIGER, E., HASEMAN, J.K., SPALDING, J., CASPARY, W., RESNICK, M., STASIEWICZ, S., ANDERSON, B. and MINOR, R. (1987). Prediction of chemical carcinogenicity in rodents from in vitro genotoxicity studies. Science 236:933–941.

Received March 7, 1988
Accepted March 24, 1988

PHYSIOLOGICAL PHARMACOKINETIC MODELS: SOME ASPECTS OF THEORY, PRACTICE AND POTENTIAL

RICHARD W. D'SOUZA* AND HAROLD BOXENBAUM†

***Miami Valley Laboratories
Procter and Gamble Company
Cincinnati, Ohio**

**†Merrell Dow Research Institute
Cincinnati, Ohio**

Models are intellectual constructs that pattern selected relationships among the elements of one system to correspond in some way to elements of a second system. In pharmacokinetics, physiological models provide a clearly articulated, rational, explanatory basis for the integration of empirical data; they do this by partitioning the biological system into relevant components (tissues, organs, etc.) and linking them together through the circulatory system. Unlike conventional mammillary compartment models, there is a clear correspondence between model system elements and physiological entities. By virtue of their high degree of physical and biochemical relevance, these models can help provide deep insight into structure, function and mechanism. Pharmacokinetic (and potentially pharmacodynamic) response-time relationships can thus be understood in terms of interconnections and behavior of constituent subsystems. At their worst, these models provide stale or infertile views of reality and thus frustrate and alienate us with the triviality of their insights. At their best, they allow us to understand the accumulation of thought in pharmacokinetics and pharmacodynamics, and help with the integration of data and improvement of experimental design.

INTRODUCTION

A major objective of virtually all scientific experimentation is to learn as much as possible with the least amount of work, to avoid activity without insight. Realization

1. Address correspondence to: Dr. Richard W. D'Souza, Miami Valley Laboratories, Procter and Gamble Company, P.O. Box 398707, Cincinnati, OH 45239-8707.
2. Key words: modeling, physiological models, scaling.

of this goal in pharmacokinetics can obviously save time and money. In the case of animal experimentation, there is often the additional goal of substituting *in vitro* for *in vivo* tests. At a time when scientists are accused of being insensitive to the pain and suffering of other sentient beings, of relegating the welfare of animals to their arrogant self-interest, reductions in *in vivo* animal experimentation through increased uses of computer simulations, physicochemical techniques, utilization of microbial systems, tissue culture methodologies, etc. are particularly attractive. As Russell and Burch (1959) put it, our goals should be the 3 Rs of replacement, reduction and refinement.

Over the past few decades, a number of attractive *in vitro* tests have been developed in the biological sciences. In toxicology, perhaps the most popular of these are the battery of screens for potential human carcinogens (Ashby et al., 1985); these tests provide a relatively inexpensive method for testing a wide range of compounds and can help identify candidates for additional mammalian bioassay. *In vitro* tests are also becoming increasingly more popular in drug screening programs and for the evaluation of safety (Office of Technology Assessment, 1986).

Use of mathematical models for simulation purposes can also reduce the amount of *in vivo* testing. With the introduction of relatively inexpensive but sophisticated high-speed digital computers, virtually all fields of biological science now employ some forms of modeling techniques. These vary in scope from simulation of the multi-leveled regulation of the cardiovascular system (Leaning et al., 1983) to the Nobel Prize winning work on theoretical aspects of the immunological system (Jerne, 1974, 1984). The modeling of hypertension by Guyton and co-workers (Guyton, 1955; Guyton and Coleman, 1969; Guyton et al., 1972) over a 17 year span provides an excellent example of how the development and availability of sophisticated computer methodology has had a significant impact on our understanding of biological control systems. Coupled with *in vitro* and limited *in vivo* experimentation, the computer-based model offers a plethora of significant biological research opportunities. In this paper, we discuss some of these possibilities as they relate to physiological pharmaco-kinetic modeling.

BASIC PRINCIPLES

Pharmacokinetics is the study of the kinetics of absorption, distribution and elimination of exogenous substances. Since it is the interplay of the aforementioned processes that determines the temporal formation and translocation of active moieties to their sites of action, and therefore the onset, duration and extent of pharmacologic response, the utility of pharmacokinetic modeling extends to all areas of biologic research involving dose-response type relationships.

Pharmacokinetics is an old science. One of the earliest models was developed by the physician, surgeon, chemist, and "magician" Philippus Aureolus Theophrastus Bombast von Hohenheim (1493-1541), known to his followers as Paracelsus the Great. In his classic treatise on miners' disease (Rosen, 1979), Paracelsus closed with a discussion of mercurial toxicity (this was the first formal writing on occupational disease). Therapy was based on the premise that mercury could deposit in the body in a stabilized form, and that, prior to elimination, it had to be mobilized. Distribution was seen to occur mechanically, through the force of gravity. Once areas of deposition were located near the skin, corrosive plasters were applied for 2-3 weeks in order to produce an ulcer through which the mercury could be excreted. The "dead" mercury was thus "revived" for passage outside the body with the help of herb or sulphur baths. Obviously a man far ahead of his time, consider the following Paracelsian physiological model: "Now it is proper to speak further concerning the evacuation of mercurius which is not alive, and how to make it alive and apt for evacuation. Note the following concerning evacuation. Every mercurius settles in the cavities of the joints. That which passes through the backbone and the hip region falls into the knee joints or ankle points through the corresponding ligaments. In the same manner mercurius vivus passes downwards when it is placed in a trench until it finds a cataract, where it remains. Thus the knees are cataracts, also the ankle joints, the hip joints and the joints of the backbone. And sometimes it collects in the ligaments, sometimes at the bottom in the soles, as deeply as it can fall. Thus it also settles in the arms, in the cataracts of the shoulders, of the elbows and further into the wrists, sometimes it falls into the neck, sometimes out of the hollow of the corner of the eye, sometimes through the nares, frequently through the pharynx into the stomach and passes out with the stool. All this can be recognized where the things are present by means of the signs and good experience."

Through modern times, many investigators have made significant contributions to pharmacokinetic science, but it was not until Torsten Teorell, a Swedish physiologist and biophysicist, published two classic articles in 1937 that the foundations of modern pharmacokinetics were laid (Wagner, 1981). Teorell's (1937a,b) physiologically based model was comprised of five compartments representing drug depot (compound at absorption site), the circulatory system, tissue distribution sites, renally eliminated drug and biotransformed drug in tissue. This pioneering work served as the forerunner upon which most pharmacokinetic models, physiological and compartmental, have developed.

The vast majority of pharmacokinetic models used to date have been of the classical (mammillary) compartmental type. Following Riggs (1963), we define a compartment as follows: "If a substance, S, is present in a biological system in several distinguishable forms or locations, and if S passes from one form or location to another form or location at a measurable rate, then each form or location constitutes a separate compartment for S." Typically, exchange between compartments occurs at first-order rates; inputs can be varied, whereas outputs are usually characterized by either first-order or Michaelis-Menten elimination pathways. There can, of course, be numerous variations on this theme; distribution can be saturable, protein binding terms can be incorporated, etc. Although these models are conceptually simplistic, and despite the fact that they do *not* purport to accurately mimic physiological processes, they have nonetheless had a significant impact. Within a relatively short period of time (about 10 years), they have radically changed our views on clinical drug therapy and drug formulation design and testing, taking them from a trial-and-error stage to one of more rational design (see Wagner, 1971 and Gibaldi and Perrier, 1983 for reviews).

Physiological pharmacokinetic models, on the other hand, do purport to accurately reflect drug behavior in biological systems. They start either with individual organs or tissues, or they lump these into groups of like-kind or like-properties (e.g., fat, rapidly equilibrating, etc.). The "compartments" are linked in an anatomically precise fashion to one another through the circulatory system. Drug elimination can occur from any compartment. By virtue of their conformance to anatomical, physiological and biochemical realities, these models have unique advantages over classical compartment models. They can, for example, adjust for alterations in organ blood flow, protein binding, shunting, etc. Since the elemental model is applicable across virtually all mammalian species (with proper adjustments), these models tend naturally to lend themselves to interspecies extrapolation.

Our purpose here is to describe the construction of these models (without getting into mathematical considerations), review some of their characteristics, and discuss their potential in drug development and toxicity programs. In particular, we shall focus on the substitution of *in vitro* experimental methodologies for *in vivo* ones.

PHYSIOLOGICAL MODEL STRUCTURE

Figure 1 illustrates a physiological model developed by Benowitz et al. (1974a) to characterize and study lidocaine disposition in monkey and man. The tissues/organs included are those considered important for drug distribution, elimination and/or pharmacodynamic activity (hair, for example, is not included). Some groups of tissues are lumped together (slowly and rapidly equilibrating tissues). As lidocaine binding to lung was expected to result in different arterial and venous drug concentrations, and given that arterial and not venous blood is relatively homogeneous, the blood pool was divided accordingly. Drug distribution within each compartment was assumed to be perfusion rate-limited, i.e., drug mixing within the compartment was assumed to occur much more rapidly than transfer to the compartment.

In this and other physiological models, three classes of parameters/variables are required: (1) anatomic/physiologic variables like organ and tissue masses and blood flows; (2) thermodynamic (partitioning) parameters like blood/plasma free fractions and tissue-to-blood partition coefficients; and (3) biochemical/biophysical parameters like metabolic and excretion rates. Once the model is mapped-out on paper, mass-balance differential equations are written for each compartment describing

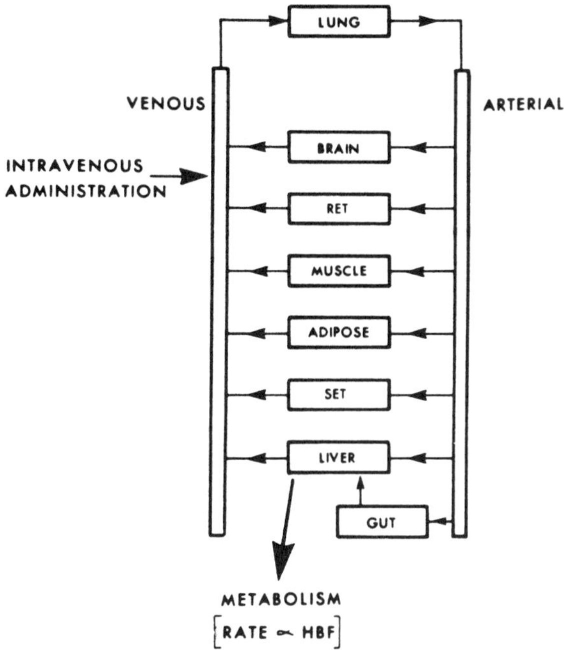

FIGURE 1. Perfusion rate-limited model used to describe lidocaine disposition kinetics in rhesus monkey and man. RET, which represents rapidly equilibrating tissues, includes heart and kidney. SET, which represents slowly equilibrating tissues, includes long bone, skull, spine, skin and chest wall. The gut is composed of the portal system (stomach, small intestine, large intestine, spleen, pancreas and mesentery). Arrows indicate the direction of blood flow. The first-order metabolism rate constant is assumed proportional to hepatic blood flow (HBF). Reproduced from Benowitz et al. (1974a) by courtesy of C. V. Mosby Co.

influx and efflux relationships. For non-eliminating, perfusion rate-limited compartments, this requires information on blood flow and binding (partitioning). For eliminating tissues, additional terms are added. These models can be adapted to accommodate such biologically relevant events as nonlinear tissue binding, Michaelis-Menten elimination, parallel organ-specific elimination, enzyme induction and inhibition, biliary recycling, diffusional resistance across cell membranes, etc. Once a set of differential equations is posited, and its accompanying parameters and variables inserted, the equations are numerically solved with the aid of a computer.

In most cases, values for tissue masses and blood flows can be obtained from compilations in the literature (see Gerlowski and Jain, 1983 for their collation in 7 mammalian species). When not available, values may be determined experimentally, scaled allometrically or simulated (trial-and-error) with the model. Binding (partitioning) parameters can be measured either by *in vivo* or *in vitro* methods. In the former case, tissue-to-blood partition coefficients may be measured at steady-state (as for example by Benowitz et al., 1974a) or during terminal exponential disposition (as for example by Harris and Gross, 1975). Although partition coefficients (ratios of tissue concentration to venous outflow blood concentration) are constant in linear, perfusion rate-limited systems, the aforementioned methods of estimation do not always provide the same answer (Chen and Gross, 1979). *In vitro* methodologies employing body fluids, isolated cell preparations, tissue homogenates, etc. have also been developed; they generally employ either equilibrium dialysis (Igari et al., 1982; Lin et al., 1982a), ultrafiltration (Kurz and Fichtl, 1983) or, for volatile substances, vial equilibration (Sato and Nakajima, 1979). In general, reasonable correlations have been observed between *in vivo* and *in vitro* values for a number of compounds (in rabbits) encompassing a broad array of physicochemical properties (Schuhmman et al., 1987). However, problems have been noted; aside from muscle, *in vitro* and *in vivo* values for cationic drugs did not relate well to one another.

In the estimation of urinary and biliary elimination parameter values, the customary procedure is to relate *in vivo* blood concentrations to rates of urinary/biliary excretion. In linear systems in which metabolism occurs within a single organ and is the only elimination pathway, metabolic clearance may be estimated by conventional methods. Benowitz et al. (1974a), for example, divided steady-state drug infusion rate by blood concentration to determine lidocaine clearance in monkeys. For volatile compounds, Andersen and co-workers (Andersen et al., 1980; Gargas et al., 1986) developed an interesting *in vivo* "gas uptake" approach utilizing a recirculating inhalation chamber. Through measurement of the decline of drug concentration in ambient air, this system can even help differentiate contributions from parallel elimination pathways. Metabolism rates can also be measured using *in vitro* techniques; these include isolated hepatocytes and other cells, supernatant fractions, microsomes, purified enzyme preparations, crude homogenates, cytosolic fractions, tissue slices, etc. Wilkinson (1987) has provided a cogent analysis of the state-of-the-art prediction of *in vivo* parameters from *in vitro* studies. A multispecies model developed for methylene chloride (Anderson et al., 1987) utilized both *in vivo* gas uptake and relative liver/lung enzymatic activities determined *in vitro*.

MODEL UTILITY

Physiological Models for Chemotherapeutic Agents. Perhaps the greatest potential for physiological models resides in the area of anti-cancer drug therapy, in the selective targeting of chemotherapeutic agents. By maximizing drug concentration at the tumor site, while keeping exposure elsewhere at a minimum, the drug's therapeutic index may be enhanced (*vide infra*).

The first anti-cancer compound to be modeled physiologically was methotrexate (see Bischoff, 1975 for a review). In rodents, this drug undergoes extensive and complex biliary recycling. To adequately fit model equations to the data, Bischoff et al. (1971) employed a rather elaborate series of discrete gut compartments with distinct transfer rate constants and lag times. This was done to "provide a smooth response" in the characterization of the data (given the complexities of biliary secretion and reabsorption). Further work on methotrexate (Dedrick et al., 1973) indicated membrane resistance in transport to bone marrow, spleen and small intestine.

Since this pioneering work, physiological models have been developed for almost a dozen chemotherapeutic agents (see Gerlowski and Jain, 1983 for a review). One good example is the model developed by Lutz et al. (1977) for actinomycin-D, an agent used for testicular tumors. In dogs, this compound exhibits diffusion resistance in its transport to testicular cells. Consequently, drug concentration profiles in testes do not parallel blood concentrations (see Fig. 2). By modeling both blood and tumor site concentration-time profiles (in a scale-up to man), dosage schedules could be tailored to achieve desired profiles in testes and/or plasma.

Another example of the application of physiological models to chemotherapeutic agents is the work by Dedrick et al. (1978) indicating that direct peritoneal administration should be an effective means of drug delivery in the treatment of ovarian cancer.

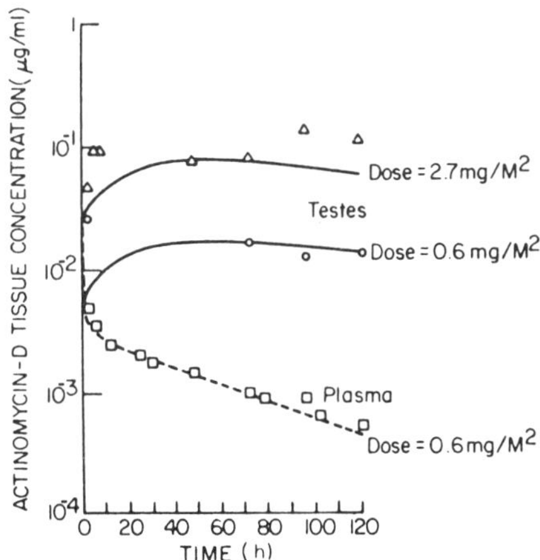

FIGURE 2. Actinomycin-D concentrations in plasma (one dose level only) and testes (two dose levels) following intravenous administration to beagle dogs. Experimentally measured points and model predictions (lines) are illustrated. A membrane-resistance model characterizing uptake by the testes was used for the simulation. Note that concentrations in the testes do not parallel those in plasma. Redrawn from Lutz et al. (1977) by courtesy of the Williams and Wilkins Company.

This conclusion is based both on the observation that ovarian tumors tend to be localized in the peritoneum and the fact that peritoneal clearance of certain chemotherapeutic agents is considerably less than blood clearance. Simulations from physiological models could aid in the design of devices (release characteristics) for regional drug delivery; the goal would be to improve the drug's therapeutic index by maximizing concentrations at tumor sites while minimizing exposure elsewhere. In addition to site-specific implantation, regional delivery of blood-borne agents to tumor sites is beginning to receive considerable attention (Molnar et al., 1984; Dedrick, 1986).

Physiological Models for Other Clinical Applications. Aside from anti-cancer compounds, drug groups studied using physiological models include antibiotics, anesthetics, metals and ions, and anticonvulsants (see Gerlowski and Jain, 1983 for other groups). Unlike conventional multicompartmental mammillary models, physiological models have the ability to simulate profiles in pathophysiological conditions. The lidocaine model illustrated in Fig. 1, for example, was used (Benowitz et al., 1974b) to investigate the effects of hemorrhagic shock and sympathomimetic drug administration on the disposition of lidocaine. The results indicated, at least in monkeys, that isoproterenol administration during shock increases lidocaine clearance (decreases plasma levels), whereas norepinephrine has the opposite effect. In both cases, the mechanism through which the sympathomimetics exerted their effects was through alteration of hepatic blood flow; in monkeys and humans, lidocaine is avidly extracted by the liver, and its clearance is therefore proportional to hepatic blood flow.

In another example, Tsuji et al. (1983) developed a generalized model for beta-lactam antibiotic disposition; properly adapted (scaled to humans), it could be used for a variety of purposes (simulating tissue/organ concentration profiles, investigating the impact of disease-induced physiological alterations, dose scheduling and optimization, etc.).

Physiological Models in Toxicology and Cancer Risk Assessment. Application of physiological modeling in these areas has received considerable attention over the past few years. In many instances, the primary goal has been to relate toxicity, cancer incidence, etc. to target-organ active moiety concentration-time profiles, cumulative amount formed, etc. Once modeled in animals, the trick usually is to extrapolate both the model and the toxic response to man. Although, at the present time, numerous models have been developed in animals, few of these have been scaled-up to acquire knowledge about humans. As is true in virtually all fields of scientific inquiry and endeavor, progress is achieved slowly. Presently, physiological modelers are struggling both with the problem of adding realistic assumptions in their procedures for extrapolation from animal to man while at the same time trying to keep their models manageable (as simple as possible). It is only now that physiological models are beginning to assimilate information from knowledge bases containing incomplete and/or contradictory information. A physiological model is not the repository of all wisdom, and many of the profound questions confronting toxicologists today go far afield or well beyond the realm of physiological model imaging. In using physiological models, we must avoid what Alfred North Whitehead termed the "fallacy of misplaced concreteness," the blunder of mistaking partial truth for the whole; rather we must adopt a healthy pluralism, accepting ambiguity while not despairing that we haven't gotten the whole of the truth (Schwartz and Wiggins, 1985).

Consider a few examples in the modeling of toxic agents. King et al. (1983) developed a physiological model in mice, rats and monkeys for 2,3,7,8-tetrachlorodibenzofuran, an environmental pollutant. Analogously, Lutz et al. (1984) characterized the disposition of several polychlorinated biphenyls in mouse, rat, dog and monkey. A physiological model for methylene chloride in mice and rats was developed (Angelo and Pritchard, 1984; Andersen et al., 1987) and used to investigate how dosing variables (vehicle and route of administration) affected the time course of concentration at potentially critical toxic sites. Andersen et al. (1987) simulated concentration-time profiles of the presumed methylene chloride carcinogenic metabolite (glutathione conjugate) in liver and lung tissue of mice, rats, hamsters and humans (tumor incidence in mice correlated well with cumulative amount of methylene chloride metabolized by the glutathione pathway). The model employed assumed first-order glutathione (GSH) conjugation in parallel with Michaelis-Menten mixed function oxidation (occurring in both liver and lung). Figure 3 illustrates relationships between methylene chloride concentration exposures/dose rates and glutathione conjugate formation rates in livers of mice and humans. Note how the model predicts an abrupt increase in slopes at the higher doses; this occurs because, as mixed function oxidation becomes saturated, a larger fraction of the dose is converted to the glutathione conjugate. The point being made here (see Fig. 3) is that metabolism/formation rates observed at higher dose-rates, and consequently the associated tumor rates, should not be extrapolated to lower dose-rates without detailed qualitative and quantitative characterization of elimination pathways; an ancillary point being made, of course, is that physiological models provide this kind of information. Model simulations also helped explain why mice developed more tumors following inhalation exposure than from drinking water administration (2000 ppm inhalation exposure produced a 56-123 fold greater amount of glutathione conjugation than did 250 mg/kg/day drinking water exposure; the total tumor incidence from drinking water was 8% compared to 63% from inhalation exposure). The physiological model was used to extrapolate target tissue glutathione conjugate doses to man; on the basis of simulations, it was suggested that methylene chloride possessed a 50-210-fold lower carcinogenic potential than had previously been thought based on estimates from more conventional models. This was the first time that a physiological pharmacokinetic model was used in a major way to project risk in humans based on data from animals. At the present time, however, neither this model nor virtually any other risk assessment model can help explain why Syrian golden hamsters (who also form glutathione conjugate) exposed to 3500 ppm methylene chloride for 6 hours/day (5 days/week) did not show a tumorigenic response at any site (Burek et al., 1984); quite the contrary,

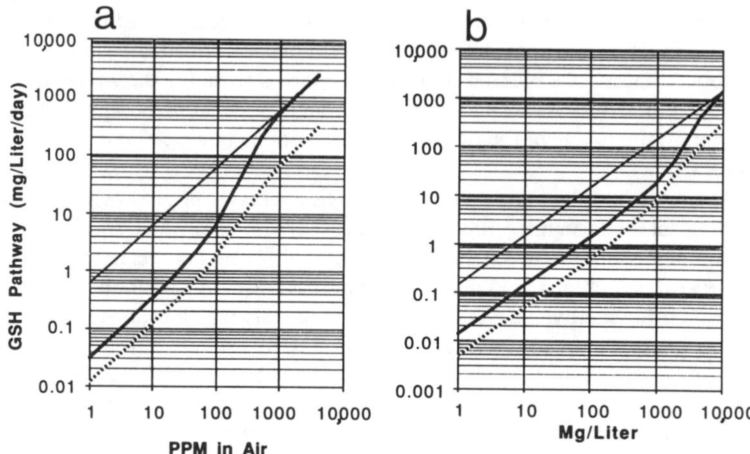

FIGURE 3. Predicted relationships between methylene chloride exposure in mice and humans and rate of hepatic formation of presumed carcinogenic metabolite (glutathione (GSH) conjugate). Exposures were assumed to occur either by inhalation (6 hours/day at the indicated ppm air concentrations) or through the drinking water (at the specified mg/liter concentrations). Physiological model predictions in mice are indicated by the heavy solid lines, whereas those in humans are shown with heavy dotted lines. By way of comparison, the lighter solid lines illustrate predictions based on linear extrapolation from data at the highest dose-rates. Note that this latter method predicts much greater formation rates than calculated from the physiological model. Reproduced from Andersen et al. (1987) by courtesy of Academic Press, Inc.

exposed animals were healthier than controls and lived longer lives (this latter observation probably results from a phenomenon termed longevity hormesis, i.e., paradoxical life-prolongation by relatively low doses of otherwise toxic agents (Neafsey, 1987)).

In an analogous manner, D'Souza et al. (1987) developed a physiologically based risk assessment model for ethylene dichloride in animals and man. In later work (D'Souza et al., 1988), the model was expanded to characterize glutathione depletion, resynthesis and "rebounding" (overshooting of control glutathione levels) in various tissues of mice and rats. Physiological models have also been applied to perchloroethylene (Travis, 1987), carbon tetrachloride (Paustenbach et al., 1987) and vinylidine chloride (D'Souza and Andersen, 1988). In this latter study, the physiological model was able to integrate and reconcile apparently disparate data between laboratories. It also helped explain observed relationships between administered dose and acute mortality.

Judging from recent publications (*vide supra*) and workshops (e.g., National Academy of Sciences, 1987), one would anticipate that physiological models will assume an increasing role as part of the risk assessment process. More than pharmacokineticists, toxicologists and their ideological brethren are adopting physiological models "to confront the established results of one region of science with the unsolved problems of another" (Beckner, 1959). In one recent paper (Conolly, 1987), for example, a physiological model was employed with a two-stage carcinogenicity model in order to simulate organ-specific accumulation of cellular mutations.

Biological Models in Teratology. To better understand risk to the human fetus, physiological animal models have been used to investigate maternal-fetal drug transfer. Olanoff and Anderson (1980), for example, developed a composite physiological model for mother and fetus in rats (see Fig. 4) and used it to study tetracycline absorption and disposition (tetracycline levels were experimentally determined in maternal, fetal and placental tissues). In order to accommodate fetal growth into the model, the fetal side of the blood flow circuit had compartment mass and blood flow variables varying as a function of time.

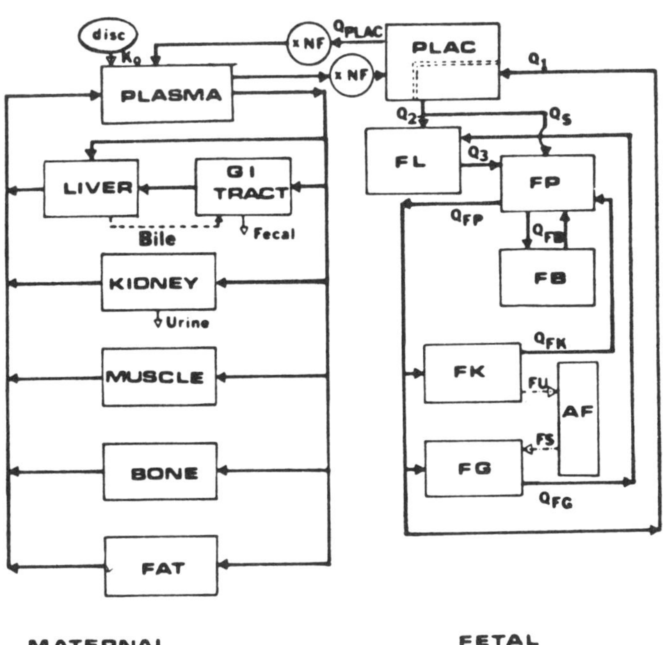

FIGURE 4. A perfusion rate-limited physiological model used to characterize tetracycline pharmacokinetics in the pregnant rat. Note that the mother and fetus are linked both anatomically and physiologically. Refer to the original reference for a description of the model and a key to the symbols (Olanoff and Anderson (1980)). Reproduced by courtesy of The Plenum Publishing Co.

As opioids are used clinically and abusively during human pregnancy, studies were conducted to gain insight into placental transport for this class of drugs. Gabrielsson and Paalzow (1983) developed a physiological model to investigate morphine disposition in pregnant rats. To be consistent with experimental data, diffusion rate-limited transport across the placenta was incorporated into the model. A similarly constructed rat model was also developed for methadone (Gabrielsson et al., 1985). Following scale-up to humans, the investigators were able to simulate methadone concentrations in maternal venous blood, maternal brain, and fetus following multiple dose oral methadone administration (once daily dosing) to the mother.

INTERSPECIES SCALING OF PHYSIOLOGICAL MODELS

The terms "scaling" and "scale-up," borrowed from the chemical engineering literature, refer to the process of extrapolation of information and knowledge gained from one system and applying it to the design or understanding of another (Dedrick, 1973). Biological scaling, as defined by Schmidt-Nielsen (1984), deals "with the structural and functional consequences of changes in size or scale among otherwise similar organisms." In engineering terms, Sjenitzer (1957) has identified four fundamental scaling types: (1) increasing the number of identical units; (2) maintaining design and function while increasing size; (3) alteration of the flow scheme; and (4) selection of different equipment. In biological systems, and consequently in scaling physiological models, all 4 scaling types have been employed. A rat has more nephrons than a mouse (type 1 scaling). On the other hand, design and function are quite similar between the two species (type 2 scaling). Blood flow rates and tissue/organ sizes are species-dependent (type 3 scaling). And whereas a mouse might eliminate intact drug through biliary excretion, a human may excrete drug predominantly in urine or metabolize it (type 4 scaling). From a functional perspective, "interspecies pharmacokinetic scaling may be viewed [simply] as any operation that produces an orderly pharmacokinetic pattern among species" (Boxenbaum and Ronfeld, 1983). Operationally, this usually translates into predicting kinetic behavior in one species (frequently man) based on data from another.

In physiological modeling, the first thing that need be considered is whether or not to structurally alter the model, to account for anatomical differences between species. Humans, for example, have a gall bladder which is not present in rats. Next, anatomic and physiologic variables (organ sizes, blood flows, etc.) need be adjusted. A 200 gram rat has about 7% body fat, compared to 20% in a 70 kg human. In most circumstances, data can be abstracted from tabulations published in the literature. If not, allometric power functions can frequently be employed. Figure 5 illustrates the use of power functions to chracterize relationships between liver size-body size as well as hepatic blood flow-body size. Calder's excellent book (1984) provides a particularly rich source of data.

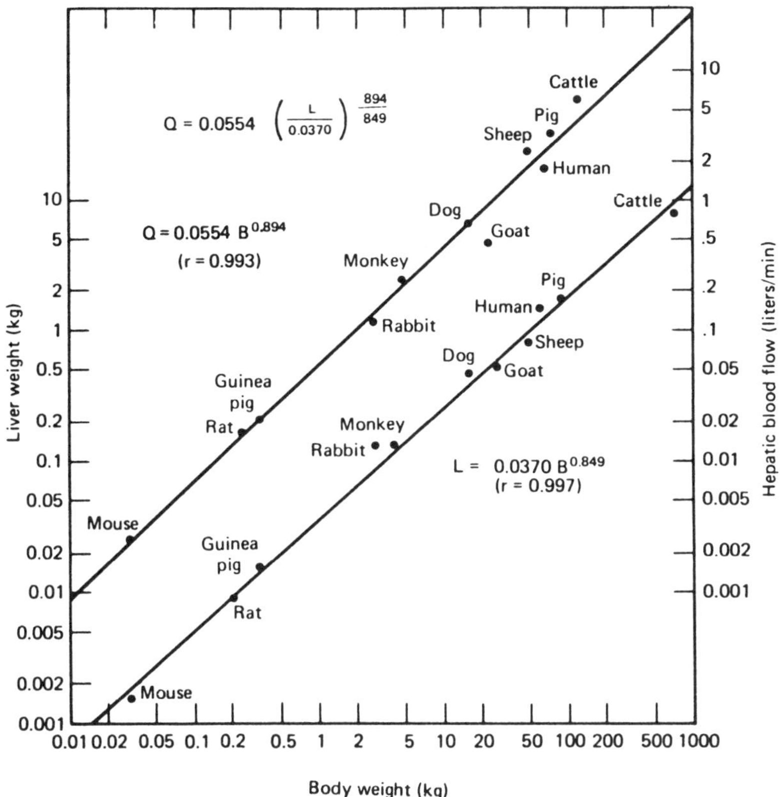

FIGURE 5. Liver weight (L) and hepatic blood flow (Q) in terrestrial mammals as a function of body weight (B). The linear relationships observed on the double logarithmic grid are consistent with simple power functions (allometric relationships) for both Q and L. Reproduced from Boxenbaum (1980) by courtesy of The Plenum Publishing Co.

Adjustments for variations in anatomic and physiologic variables are relatively simple. Difficulties really arise when extrapolating thermodynamic (partitioning) and biochemical/biophysical parameters. Blood and tissue binding parameters frequently differ across species. If at all possible, it is desirable to experimentally determine blood and tissue binding parameters for all species of interest. In the case of man, however, given the unavailability of human cadaver tissue, this is generally impractical. Therefore, the usual procedure is to use tissue partition coefficients from animals (referenced to total blood concentration). In the case of perfusion rate-limited distribution, a more rational approach would be to correct these partition coefficients to unbound blood drug concentration. At the very least, binding to human blood components should be determined experimentally.

In scaling biochemical/biophysical parameters, there are two options. The first (and best) is to determine these experimentally in all species being studied. If this is not possible, as for example with very toxic substances in humans, these parameters can either be scaled (power functions are the most common relationships) or empirically estimated by trial-and-error. Although the latter approach need sometimes be resorted to, it is an anathema. The primary purpose of physiological modeling is to accurately and realistically depict and characterize pharmacokinetic events within the organism. Expediency is not a methodological exemplar easily swallowed by physiological modelers; after all, this is what differentiates them from conventional pharmacokineticists! Consequently, the more commonly used approach is that of interspecies extrapolation, and investigators freely arrogate to themselves considerable latitude in this respect. This may entail, for example, *a priori* assignment of an allometric exponent (usually on the order of 0.25 or 0.75), calculation of the corresponding coefficient in the same single species, and extrapolation of the entire relationship to another species. Although beyond the scope of this present discussion, allometric extrapolation of drug metabolism parameters to man is extremely tenuous (in contradistinction to extrapolation of anatomic, physiologic and other biochemical variables in man, which are usually quite reliable). Evolutionary adaptation (fitness for an environment), and its mechanism of natural selection, has placed considerable limits on what can be or is most likely to be found anatomically, physiologically and biochemically (this is sometimes referred to as biological design). In characterizing this regularity, the simple allometric equation (power function) has extraordinary predictive value, but not necessarily when it comes to deducing drug metabolism rates in man, particularly when oxidation reactions are involved (Yates and Kugler, 1986; Boxenbaum, 1984, 1986; Boxenbaum and D'Souza, 1988a,b). Using the simple allometric function for animals and applying it to man, one predicts a value for antipyrine intrinsic clearance of unbound drug approximately 7-fold greater than that found experimentally (Boxenbaum, 1980).

There are numerous examples of scaling from one species to another, so we can only describe a few here. The lidocaine model depicted in Fig. 1 was one of the first models scaled to humans. The human arterial blood concentration-time profile was well predicted using experimentally estimated partition coefficients from monkeys. Human tissue masses, blood flows and the hepatic extraction ratio was obtained from the literature. The study by Lin et al. (1982b) is particularly interesting, since it scaled ethoxybenzamide pharmacokinetics from rat to rabbit based solely on *in vitro* data. Andersen et al. (1987) used a combination of scaling approaches for their methylene chloride model in mice, rats, hamsters and man. Allometry was used for some tissue masses and blood flows, *in vivo* "gas uptake" was used to help characterize overall metabolism rate and *in vitro* techniques were employed for determination of partition coefficients as well as relative lung:liver metabolic enzymatic activities.

DISCUSSION

Physiological pharmacokinetic models offer a unified, methodological approach for studying the behavior of chemicals in living systems. Although used extensively for a variety of diverse applications, their full potential is far from being realized. Two possible explanations are offered. First, these models have only recently gone through an expansive developmental stage; much of the basic information and experimental methodologies (including validation) required for routine application are only now becoming available. This process has naturally been time consuming and expensive, and relatively few laboratories have been involved. This situation should not persist in the future; several good review articles have now appeared, anatomic and blood flow variables have been collected for several species and *in vitro* methodologies have been developed for estimation of partition coefficients, and, in some situations, metabolism rates. Andersen and co-workers[a] have already made experimental determinations of partition coefficients and metabolism rates for over 50 volatile compounds in rats. Physiological disposition of these compounds can now be simulated in a variety of species without additional laboratory work. Additionally, a generalized model for the disposition of volatile compounds is available on floppy disks for use on personal computers (Clewell and Anderson, 1986). A second and somewhat ironic reason that physiological models have not been fully exploited is that those biological scientists who would most benefit from their application have been frightened away by the mathematics. This may have been due in part to their lack of experience with the mathematical techniques as well as unfamiliarity with software for dynamic simulation modeling (a number of excellent simulation packages are now available, some of which are described by Menzel et al. (1987)). Physiological modelers must also share some of the criticism; far too many articles have been unnecessarily abstruse, and many biologists feel alienated. As Alfred North Whitehead noted, it is as though "the concrete world has slipped through meshes of the scientific net." Modelers must stop confounding us with dense mathematical arguments and other obfuscations. The greatest American scientist (J. Willard Gibbs) has told us that "the whole is simpler than the sum of its parts," but it is clear that not all have taken heed.

The physiological approach offers an abundance of possibilities for the establishment of model structure and function. Heuristically, the modeler can temporarily suspend exactness and vigor and play "what if?" games. Much can be learned from failure; as commonly appreciated (Sacher, 1970; Kaplan, 1964; Box, 1979; Yates, 1978), good models serve useful purposes when they fail just as when they succeed. Psychologically, models may be most appealing when they succeed, but they are logically strongest when they fail—you know to reject your hypothesis (Yates, 1978). Good symbolic, conceptual analogies (i.e., physiological models) allow for systematic

---

[a]Melvin E. Andersen, Personal communication.

exploitation of failure (Kaplan, 1964). Systematic deviations between data and model predictions/simulations often suggest alternative strategies, leading to new tentative models.

As an example, Andersen and colleagues (Andersen et al., 1986; Clewell and Andersen, 1987; D'Souza et al., 1987, 1988) noted that their rodent model for halogenated hydrocarbon disposition did not adequately characterize allyl chloride or ethylene dichloride disposition. By simulating a number of possible model alternatives, they hypothesized (and later experimentally demonstrated) that these compounds alter their own metabolism rates by co-substrate (glutathione) depletion.

One can envision many future uses of physiological models. Chronic cancer bioassay studies are conducted with little or no information about disposition. For methylene chloride and ethylene dichloride, physiological models have clearly demonstrated that bioassays have been conducted at doses at which detoxifying enzymes are saturated, doses nowhere near those that humans would normally receive. Extrapolation of risk (excess cancer incidence) from animal to man should consider pharmacokinetic factors of this nature. The aforementioned studies also demonstrated that relative "target organ doses" of toxic moieties (to liver and lung) were highly dependent upon route of administration (oral vs. inhalation).

Physiological models can obviously provide useful information regarding dosing regimens, routes of administration and inter-species extrapolation. They can also be used to explore different mechanistic possibilities (hypothesis testing) when anomalous results are obtained. In teratology testing, physiological models can sometimes be used to determine fetal target organ concentrations (relative to maternal exposure). They can thus provide useful information for establishing realistic concentrations of potential teratogens during *in vitro* testing. Presently, for lack of other reasonable criteria, peak maternal plasma concentrations are sometimes used; frequently, even less meaningful standards are employed, e.g., a mg/kg maternal dose may be equated to a mg/liter fetal exposure. Physiological models can also be used to study fetal growth patterns (Ranson, 1981).

In drug development, physiological models might help select candidates for testing in humans. It is not uncommon to have several pre-clinical compounds, all with pharmacodynamic activity. A global physiological model might help provide insight into why one compound is more or less active than another, for example, why a particular compound with good *in vitro* activity only has modest *in vivo* activity (first pass effects, diffusion rate-limited entry to active sites, etc.). This information could also be used to help design and interpret results of short or long-term toxicity studies. With refinement, the model might also be scaled-up to man to help optimize therapy (routes of administration, dosing regimens, etc.).

Given newer developments, it will be easier than ever for biologists to translate observations and descriptions of biological processes into clear mathematical expressions and simulations. In exploiting the new technology, the investigator must be careful not to lead himself or his colleagues "from sets of more or less plausible but entirely arbitrary assumptions to precisely stated but irrelevant theoretical conclusions" (Leontief, 1982). Experimental verification is important. There is also the all-too-human tendency to force-fit models to data; as one anonymous commentator put it: "... almost any set of data, if sufficiently badgered, can be exhausted into submission."

"To know the world, one must construct it" (Cesare Pavese). Physiological model building holds great promise for biological research, be it for heuristic simulation aimed at elucidating structure and/or function, optimization of dosage regimens, etc. For the modeler who is properly focused, these models can be used to streamline and/or minimize laboratory investigation, decrease experimental costs and manpower, reduce experimental animal numbers and, of course, advance scientific knowledge. But even if, deep down, lingering doubts about the fertility of these models persist, bear in mind that "a clash of doctrines is not a disaster—it is an opportunity" (A. N. Whitehead).

ACKNOWLEDGEMENT

The authors wish to express their appreciation to Dr. Melvin E. Andersen for his helpful comments, suggestions and criticisms.

REFERENCES

ASHBY, J., DeSERRES, F.J., DRAPER, M., ISHIDATE, M., MARGOLIN, B.H., MATTER, B.E. and SHELBY, M.D., eds. (1985). Progress in Mutation Research—Evaluation of Short Term Tests for Carcinogens, Elsevier, New York.

ANDERSEN, M.E., CLEWELL III, H.J., GARGAS, M.L. and CONOLLY, R.B. A physiological pharmacokinetic model for hepatic glutathione (GSH) depletion by inhaled halogenated hydrocarbons. Toxicologist **6**:148 (1986).

ANDERSEN, M.E., CLEWELL III, H.J., GARGAS, M.L., SMITH, F.A. and REITZ, R.H. (1987). Physiologically based pharmacokinetics and the risk assessment process for methylene chloride. Toxicol. Appl. Pharmacol. **87**:185–205.

ANDERSEN, M.E., GARGAS, M.L., JONES, R.A. and JENKINS, JR., L.J. (1980). Determination of the kinetic constants for metabolism of inhaled toxicants in vivo using gas uptake measurements. Toxicol. Appl. Pharmacol. **54**:100–116.

ANGELO, M.J. and PRITCHARD, A.B. (1984). Simulations of methylene chloride pharmacokinetics using a physiologically based model. Reg. Toxicol. Pharmacol. **4**:329–339.

BECKNER, M. (1959). The Biological Way of Thought, p. 52. Columbia University Press, New York.

BENOWITZ, N., FORSYTH, R.P., MELMON, K.L. and ROWLAND, M. (1974a). Lidocaine disposition kinetics in monkey and man. I. Prediction by a perfusion model. Clin. Pharmacol. Therap. **16**:87–98.

BENOWITZ, N., FORSYTH, R.P., MELMON, K.L. and ROWLAND, M. (1974b). Lidocaine disposition kinetics in monkey and man. II. Effects of hemorrhage and sympathomimetic drug administration. Clin. Pharmacol. Therap. **16**:99–109.

BISHOFF, K.B. (1975). Some fundamental considerations of the applications of pharmacokinetics to cancer chemotherapy. Cancer Chemother. Rep. **59**:777–793.

BISHOFF, K.B., DEDRICK, R.L., ZAHARKO, D.S. and LONGSTRETCH, J.A. (1971). Methotrexate pharmacokinetics. J. Pharm. Sci. **8**:1128–1133.

BOX, G.E.P. (1979). Robustness in the strategy of scientific model building. In: Robustness in Statistics (R.L. Launer and G.N. Wilkinson, eds.), pp. 201–236, Academic Press, New York.

BOXENBAUM, H. (1980). Interspecies variation in liver weight, hepatic blood flow, and antipyrine intrinsic clearance: Extrapolation of data to benzodiazepines and phenytoin. J. Pharmacokin. Biopharm. **8**:165–176.

BOXENBAUM, H. (1984). Interspecies pharmacokinetic scaling and the evolutionary-comparative paradigm. Drug Metab. Rev. **15**:1071–1121.

BOXENBAUM, H. (1986). Time concepts in physics, biology, and pharmacokinetics. J. Pharm. Sci. **75**:1053–1062.

BOXENBAUM, H. and D'SOUZA, R. (1988a). Physiological models, allometry, neoteny, space-time, and pharmacokinetics. In: Pharmacokinetics: Mathematical and Statistical Approaches (A. Pecile and A. Rescigno, eds.), Plenum Press, New York, in press.

BOXENBAUM, H. and D'SOUZA, R. (1988b). Interspecies pharmacokinetic scaling: Reductionist and allometric paradigms. In: Proceedings of the 47th International Congress of Pharmaceutical Sciences of F.I.P. (D. D. Breimer, ed.), Elsevier, Amsterdam, in press.

BOXENBAUM, H. and RONFIELD, R. (1983). Interspecies pharmacokinetic scaling and the Dedrick plots. Am. J. Physiol. **245**:R768–R775.

BUREK, J.D., NITSCHKE, K.D., BELL, T.J., WACKERLE, D.L., CHILDS, R.C., BEYER, J.E., DITTENBER, D.A., RAMPY, L.W. and McKENNA, M.J. (1984). Methylene chloride: A two-year inhalation toxicity and oncogenicity study in rats and hamsters. Fund. Appl. Toxicol. **4**:30–47.

CALDER III, W.A. (1984). Size, Function, and Life History. Harvard University Press, Cambridge.

CHEN, G.H-S. and GROSS, J.F. (1979). Estimation of tissue-to-plasma partition coefficients in physiologic pharmacokinetic models. J. Pharmacokinet. Biopharm. **7**:117–125.

CLEWELL III, H.J. and ANDERSEN, M.E. (1986). A multiple dose route physiological pharmacokinetic model for volatile chemicals using ACSL-PC. In: Languages for Continuous Systems Simulation (F.D. Cellier, ed.), pp. 95–101, Society of Computer Simulation Publications, San Diego; floppy disks available through Mitchell & Gauthier, Concord, Mass.

CLEWELL, III, H.J. and ANDERSEN, M.E. (1987). Dose, species, and route extrapolation using physiologically based pharmacokinetic models. In: Pharmacokinetics in Risk Assessment: Drinking Water and Health, Vol. 8, pp. 159–182. National Academy Press, Washington, DC.

CONOLLY, R.B., REITZ, R.H. and ANDERSEN, M.E. (1987). Mutation accumulation: A biologically based mathematical model of chronic cytotoxicant exposure. In: Pharmacokinetics in Risk Assessment: Drinking Water and Health, Vol. 8, pp. 273–285. National Academy Press, Washington, DC.

DEDRICK, R.L. (1973). Animal scale-up. J. Pharmacokinet. Biopharm. **1**:435–460.

DEDRICK, R.L. (1986). Interspecies scaling of regional drug delivery. J. Pharm. Sci. **75**:1047–1052.

DEDRICK, R.L., MYERS, C.E., BUNGAY, P.M. and DEVITA, JR., V.T. (1978). Pharmacokinetic rationale for peritoneal drug administration in the treatment of ovarian cancer. Cancer Treat. Rep. **62**:1–9.

DEDRICK, R.L., ZAHARKO, D.S. and LUTZ, R.J. (1973). Transport and binding of methotrexate in vivo. J. Pharm. Sci. **62**:882–890.

D'SOUZA, R.W. and ANDERSEN, M.E. (1988). Physiologically based pharmacokinetic model for vinylidine chloride. Toxicol. Appl. Pharmacol., in press.

D'SOUZA, R.W., FRANCIS, W.R. and ANDERSEN, M.E. (1988). Physiological model for tissue glutathione depletion and resynthesis following ethylene dichloride exposure. J. Pharmacol. Exp. Therap., in press.

D'SOUZA, R.W., FRANCIS, W.R., BRUCE, R.D. and ANDERSEN, M.E. (1987). Physiologically based pharmacokinetic model for ethylene dichloride, and its application in risk assessment. In: Pharmacokinetics in Risk Assessment: Drinking Water and Health, Vol. 8, pp. 286–301. National Academy Press, Washington, DC.

GABRIELSSON, J.L., JOHANSSON, P., BONDESSON, U. and PAALZOW, L.K. (1985). Analysis of methadone disposition in the pregnant rat by means of a physiological flow model. J. Pharmacokinet. Biopharm. **13**:355–372.

GABRIELSSON, J.L. and PAALZOW, L.K. (1983). A physiological pharmacokinetic model for morphine disposition in the pregnant rat. J. Pharmacokinet. Biopharm. **11**:147–163.

GARGAS, M.L., ANDERSEN, M.E. and CLEWELL, III, H.J. (1986). A physiologically based simulation approach for determining metabolic constants from gas uptake data. Toxicol. Appl. Pharmacol. **86**:341–352.

GERLOWSKI, L.E. and JAIN, R.K. (1983). Physiologically based pharmacokinetic modeling: Principles and applications. J. Pharm. Sci. **72**:1103–1127.

GIBALDI, M. and PERRIER, D. (1982). Pharmacokinetics. Marcel Dekker, New York.

GUYTON, A.C. (1955). Determination of cardiac output by equating venous return curves with cardiac response curves. Physiol. Rev. **35**:123–129.

GUYTON, A.C. and COLEMAN, T.G. (1969). Quantitative analysis of the pathophysiology of hypertension. Circ. Res. **24**:1–19.

GUYTON, A.C., COLEMAN, T.G. and GRANGER, H.J. (1972). Circulation: Overall Regulation. Ann. Rev. Physiol. **34**:13–46.

HARRIS, P.A. and GROSS, J.F. (1975). Preliminary pharmacokinetics models for adriamycin (NSC-123127). Cancer Chemother. Rep., Part I, **59**:819–825.

IGARI, Y., SUGIYAMA, Y., AWAZU, S. and HANANO, M. (1982). Comparative physiologically based pharmacokinetics of hexobarbital, phenobarbital and thiopental in the rat. J. Pharmacokinet. Biopharm. **10**:53–75.

JERNE, N.K. (1974). The immune system: A web of V-domains. Harvey Lect. **70**:93–110.

JERNE, N.K. (1984). Idiotypic networks and other preconceived ideas. Immunol. Rev. **79**:5–24.

KAPLAN, A. (1964). The Conduct of Inquiry. Chandler Publishing Co., San Francisco.

KING, F.G., DEDRICK, R.L., COLLINS, J.M., MATTHEWS, H.B. and BIRNBAUM, L.S. (1983). Physiological model for the pharmacokinetics of 2,3,7,8-tetrachlorodibenzofuran in several species. Toxicol. Appl. Pharmacol. **67**:390–400.

KURZ, H. and FICHTL, B. (1983). Binding of drugs to tissues. Drug Metab. Rev. 14:467–510.

LEANING, M.S., CARSON, E.R. and FINKELSTEIN, L. (1983). Modelling a complex biological system: the human cardiovascular system—1. Methodology and model description. Trans. Inst. Meas. Control 5:71–86.

LEONTIEF, W. (1982). Academic economics. Science 217:104, 107.

LIN, J.H., SUGIYAMA, Y., AWAZU, S. and HANANO, M. (1982a). In vitro and in vivo evaluation of the tissue-to-blood partition coefficient for physiologic pharmacokinetic models. J. Pharmacokinet. Biopharm. 10:637–647.

LIN, J.H., SUGIYAMA, Y., AWAZU, S. and HANANO, M. (1982b). Physiological pharmacokinetics of ethoxybenzamide based on biochemical data obtained in vitro as well as physiological data. J. Pharmacokin. Biopharm. 10:649–661.

LUTZ, R.J., DEDRICK, R.L., TUEY, D., SIPES, I.G., ANDERSON, M.W. and MATTHEWS, H.B. (1984). Comparison of the pharmacokinetics of several polychlorinated biphenyls in mouse, rat, dog, and monkey by means of a physiological pharmacokinetic model. Drug Metab. Disp. 12:527–535.

LUTZ, R.J., GALBRAITH, W.M., DEDRICK, R.L., SHRAGER, R. and MELLETT, L.B. (1977). A model for the kinetics of distribution of actinomycin-D in the beagle dog. J. Pharmacol. Exp. Therap. 200:469–478.

MENZEL, D.B., WOLPERT, R.L., BOGER III, J.R. and KOOTSEY, J.M. (1987). Resources available for simulation in toxicology: Specialized computers, general software, and communication networks. In: Pharmacokinetics and Risk Assessment: Drinking Water and Health, Vol. 8, pp. 229–250. National Academy Press. Washington, DC.

MOLNAR, P., BROOTHUIS, D., BLASBERG, R., ZAHARKO, D., OWENS, E. and FENSTERMACHER, J. (1984). Regional thymidine transport and incorporation in experimental brain and subcutaneous tumors. J. Neurochem. 43:421–432.

NATIONAL ACADEMY OF SCIENCES. (1987). Pharmacokinetics in Risk Assessment: Drinking Water and Health, Vol. 8, National Academy Press, Washington, DC.

NEAFSEY, P.J. (1987). Pharmacokinetic dose-response models of mortality data from chronic toxicity studies. Dissertation for the degree of Doctor of Philosophy, University of Connecticut, Storrs, CT.

OFFICE OF TECHNOLOGY ASSESSMENT. (1986). Alternatives to Animal Use in Research, Testing, and Education. U.S. Government Printing Office, Washington, DC.

OLANOFF, L.S. and ANDERSON, J.M. (1980). Controlled release of tetracycline-III: A physiological pharmacokinetic model of the pregnant rat. J. Pharmacokinet. Biopharm. 8:599–620.

PAUSTENBACH, D.J., CLEWELL III, H.J., GARGAS, M.L. and ANDERSEN, M.E. (1987). Development of a physiologically based pharmacokinetic model for multiday inhalation of carbon tetrachloride. In: Pharmacokinetics and Risk Assessment: Drinking Water and Health, Vol. 8, pp. 312–326. National Academy Press, Washington, DC.

RANSON, R. (1981). Computers and Embryos: Models in Development Biology, John Wiley and Sons, New York.

RIGGS, D.S. (1963). The Mathematical Approach to Physiological Problems, pp. 171–172, Williams & Wilkins Co., Baltimore.

ROSEN, G. (1979). Translation and Commentary on: "On the Miners' Sickness and Other Miners' Diseases" by Theophrastus von Hohenheim, called Paracelsus. In: Four Treatises of Theophrastus von Hohenheim, called Paracelsus (H.E. Sigerist, ed.), pp. 43–126, Arno Press, New York (original copyright 1941 by Johns Hopkins Press, Baltimore).

RUSSELL, W.M.S. and BURCH, R.L. (1959). The Principles of Humane Experimental Technique. Methuen, London.

SACHER, G.A. (1970). Models from radiation toxicity data. In: Late Effects of Radiation (R.J.M. Fry, D. Grahn, M.L. Griem and J.H. Rust, eds.), Chapter X, pp. 233–244, Taylor & Francis Ltd., London.

SATO, A. and NAKAJIMA, T. (1979). Partition coefficients of some aromatic hydrocarbons and ketones in water, blood and oil. Brit. J. Ind. Med. **36**:231–234.

SCHMIDT-NIELSEN, K. (1984). Scaling: Why is Animal Size So Important? p. 7, Cambridge University Press, Cambridge.

SCHUHMANN, G., FICHTL, B. and KURZ, H. (1987). Prediction of drug distribution in vivo on the basis of in vitro binding data. Biopharm. Drug Dispos. **8**:73–76.

SCHWARTZ, M.A. and WIGGINS, O. (1985). Science, humanism, and the nature of medical practice: A phenomenological view. Persp. Biol. Med. **28**:331–361.

SJENITZER, F.; through NO AUTHOR (1957). Discussion of papers presented at the first session. In: Scaling-Up of Chemical Plant and Processes (J. M. Pirie, honorary ed.), pp. S26–S27, The Institution of Chemical Engineers, London.

TEORELL, T. (1937a). Kinetics of the distribution of substances administered to the body. I. The extravascular modes administration. Arch. Intern. Pharmacodyn. **57**:205–225.

TEORELL, T. (1937b). Kinetics of the distribution of substances administered to the body. II. The intravascular modes of administration. Arch. Intern. Pharmacodyn. **57**:226–240.

TRAVIS, C.C. (1987). Interspecies and dose-route extrapolations. In: Pharmacokinetics and Risk Assessment: Drinking Water and Health, Vol. 8, pp. 208–220. National Academy Press, Washington, DC.

TUSJI, A., YOSHIKAWA, T., NISHIDE, K., MINAMI, H., KIMURA, M., NAKA-SHIMA, E., TERASAKI, T., MIYAMOTO, E., NIGHTINGALE, C.H. and YAMANA, T. (1983). Physiologically based pharmacokinetic model for beta-lactam antibiotics I: Tissue distribution and elimination in rats. J. Pharm. Sci. **72**:1239–1251.

WAGNER, J.G. (1971). Biopharmaceutics and Relevant Pharmacokinetics. Drug Intelligence Publications, Hamilton.

WAGNER, J.G. (1981). History of Pharmacokinetics. Pharmacol. Ther. **12**:537–562.

WILKINSON, G.R. (1987). Prediction of in vivo parameters of drug metabolism and distribution from in vitro studies. In: Pharmacokinetics in Risk Assessment: Drinking Water and Health, Vol. 8, pp. 80–95. National Academy Press, Washington, DC.

YATES, F.E. (1978). Good manners in good modeling: Mathematical models and computer simulations of physiological systems. Am. J. Physiol. **234**:R159–R160.

YATES, F.E. and KUGLER, P.N. (1986). Similarity principles and intrinsic geometries: Contrasting approaches to interspecies scaling. J. Pharm. Sci. **75**:1019–1027.

Received February 11, 1988
Accepted February 22, 1988

AN OVERVIEW OF STRUCTURE-ACTIVITY RELATIONSHIPS AS AN ALTERNATIVE TO TESTING IN ANIMALS FOR CARCINOGENICITY, MUTAGENICITY, DERMAL AND EYE IRRITATION, AND ACUTE ORAL TOXICITY

KURT ENSLEIN

Health Designs, Inc.
Rochester, New York

The use of structure-activity relationships (SAR) has proven practical for the development of equations which can be used to estimate the above-listed endpoints for a large variety of chemicals. The SAR models predict these endpoints correctly in 85 to 97% of the cases and often surpass in their predictive ability the results obtainable from the equivalent biological assays.

These SAR models are being used at several levels: drug, or more generally, chemical discovery; prioritization for testing; regulatory affairs; investigation of detoxification mechanisms; and risk estimation.

*In the new compound (**discovery**) use, potential toxic effects of a set of related compounds are investigated before synthesis to select those chemicals with the lesser probabilities of producing toxic effects for further investigation, at considerable savings in research expenditure since fewer compounds need to be synthesized, and the avoidance of blind alleys. **Prioritization** for testing is used in numerous instances, such as selecting those chemicals in an environment which are most likely to have toxic effects for priority attention. SAR models are used by **regulatory** agencies to determine the possible toxic effects of chemicals for which data insufficient to render decisions have been submitted, and to gain insight into possible toxicity problems. SAR models are also used to investigate possible **metabolites**, and toxicity mechanisms due to the ability of making computer-based **structural modifications** and observing the effects on the modelled toxic endpoints. **Risk analysis***

---

1. Address correspondence to: Kurt Enslein, Health Designs, Inc., 183 East Main Street, Rochester, NY 14604.

2. Key words: acute toxicity, carcinogenicity, eye irritation, mutagenicity, skin (dermal) irritation, structure-activity relationships.

3. Abbreviation: SAR, structure activity relationship.

is a natural outgrowth of several of the above applications, and is particularly useful for SAR models of carcinogenicity.

SAR models as alternatives to animal bioassays should be used in the context of other information for the chemicals of concern. Just as bioassays and in vitro *methods have their limitations, so do SAR models. These include the sometimes limited data base on which to base an SAR model, the temptation to extrapolate beyond the confines of the model, and the noise inherent in the bioassays on which the models are based. Within these constraints SAR models have a considerable potential in reducing the number of animals used in toxicity testing.*

INTRODUCTION AND OVERVIEW

Structure-activity relationships (SAR) have been used for many years for the development and optimization of pharmaceutical and agricultural chemicals (Hansch and Leo, 1979). We have applied these principles to the development of SAR models of toxic endpoints (Enslein, 1984). These models permit the estimation of these toxic effects from the structure of chemicals which have not been bioassayed. The use of *in calculo* toxicity estimates reduces the need for *in vivo* bioassays, and thus leads to fewer animals being used in toxicological research.

The elements needed for the development of an SAR model are:

- A data base of verified assays for the endpoints in question;
- A set of parameters which describe the chemical structures so that the endpoint can be modelled in terms of these parameters;
- Statistical techniques, principally multivariate regression and discriminant analysis, for weighting these parameters in a near-optimum fashion for the explanation of the endpoint;
- Computer technology to make it all practical.

Comprehensive reviews of these requirements have been previously published (Enslein, 1984).

Toxicity estimates derived from SAR models are being used for the following types of applications:

- In compound discovery, to select for further investigation those chemicals from among a set of candidates which are less likely to have toxic effects, thus maximizing the return on research investment;
- Prioritization of chemicals of environmental concern to permit the selection of those most in need of bioassay, inasmuch as the great majority of chemicals have not been, and never will be, tested;

- Investigation of detoxification by studying the effects of modifications of the structure on the toxic effect;
- Investigation of the toxic effects of putative metabolites;
- Identification of compounds for risk assessment.

In Section II of this paper we will describe the performance characteristics of the SAR models currently included in the TOPKAT program; Section III details the steps involved in the derivation of an estimate for a Draize eye irritation score; and Section IV discusses limitations and other considerations of the applicability of these SAR models.

PERFORMANCE OF SAR MODELS

In this section, we will cover performance characteristics of the following SAR models:

- Carcinogenicity
- Mutagenicity (Ames)
- Draize skin irritation
- Draize eye irritation
- Rat oral LD50

Carcinogenicity. This model predicts the probability that a compound would be declared a rodent carcinogen if it were tested according to the 2-year NCI/NTP carcinogenesis protocol. The data ($N = 335$) for this model were derived from the following sources:

- The NCI/NTP assays as classified into nine categories by Dr. R. Griesemer (1980); Dr. Griesemer has continued the classification of NTP bioassays beyond those published in 1980;
- Food additives listed in Code of Federal Regulations 21 (CFR, 1979) which have been used for substantial periods of time and sometimes in considerable quantities, and are, at least putatively, in the absence of any evidence to the contrary, noncarcinogenic;
- Pharmaceutical chemicals for which 2-year rodent bioassays have been performed;
- Human carcinogens listed in the Fourth Annual Report on Carcinogens (USDHHS, 1985).

The discriminant equation which embodies this model results in Table 1.

Of the 335 chemicals in the data base, seven could not be classified by the equation. Of the remaining 328 chemicals, seven were classified as positive when in fact they tested negative, and three were classified as negative by the equation, when in fact they were carcinogens. This results in false positive and negative rates of 2.1% and 0.9%, respectively. The overall accuracy of the SAR model is 97% (Enslein et al., 1987a).

TABLE 1
Carcinogenicity Model Classification

Bioassay	Discriminant Equation Classification	
	Negative	Positive
Negative	217	7
Positive	3	101

These error rates are based on the chemicals which were used in the design of the model. Snapinn and Knoke (1985) have shown that the error rate obtained from a discriminant equation using the resubstitution method (i.e., estimating the error rates with the compounds used in the design of the equation) is equivalent to using an independent test sample, as long as the two classification groups are sufficiently separated in the parameter space, the number of chemicals is large enough, and a "no decision" zone is used between the two groups. In our case, this zone is represented by the probability range of 0.3 to 0.7, the "indeterminate" zone. The seven compounds which cannot be classified fall into that range.

Mutagenicity. This SAR model is based on 805 chemicals assayed by the Ames (*Salmonella typhimurium*) assay (Enslein et al., 1986/87). The bulk of the data were reviewed by panels of the EPA Gene-Tox program. These panels examine the experimental evidence for and against mutagenicity on a strain-by-strain basis, with and without liver homogenate (S9) activation, and arrive at an overall conclusion from the available evidence. While dose-response data for the assays are available for a subset of these chemicals, the SAR model is limited to determining the probability of a compound being classified as a mutagen were an Ames assay performed on it.

The performance of this equation is shown in Table 2.

Of the 805 chemicals in the data base, 53 (6.6%) could not be classified by the equation. Of the remaining 752 chemicals, the equation classified seven as positive when in fact they tested negative, and 29 as negative when in fact they were Ames mutagens. This

TABLE 2
Mutagenicity Model Classification

Bioassay	Discriminant Equation Classification	
	Negative	Positive
Negative	236	7
Positive	29	480

TABLE 3
Skin Irritation Model Data Sources

Source	Scoring Method	Number of Compounds
Research Institute of Fragrance Materials (11)	Draize	350
U.S. Army Environmental Hygiene Agency	Draize	144
Smyth et al.	10-point	63
Marhold, Institute of Hygiene	10-point	213
Other	Various	24
		794

results in false positive and negative rates of 0.9% and 3.9%, respectively. The overall accuracy of the SAR model is 95.2%.

Note that it is also possible to express these misclassification rates in terms of the total negative or positive compounds. For example, there are 243 Ames negative compounds in the model, of which seven were misclassified; this results in a (conditional) misclassification rate of $7/243 = 2.9\%$. Similarly, the conditional misclassification rate for the positives is $29/509 = 5.7\%$. Whether one uses the absolute or conditional misclassification rate depends on the application of the estimate.

Rabbit Skin Irritation. This SAR model estimates the probability that exposure to a chemical would result in one of four possible degrees of skin irritation, rated according to the Draize scale (Draize et al., 1944), i.e., none, mild, moderate, or severe. The data were mostly obtained from the open literature. While it would be reasonable to assume that the bulk of the data were the results of Draize assays, in fact many of the data were scored on a scale due to the Smyth et al. group (1944, 1948, 1949, 1951, 1954, 1962; Weil and Scala 1971). This same scoring method was then used by Marhold at the Institute of Hygiene (Marhold, 1972) in Czechoslovakia. The 10-point scores were then rescaled in order to fit them into the Draize four-level scheme. The sources of data and the number of compounds contributed by each are given in Table 3.

Of these 794 compounds, 786 were used in the development of the skin irritation estimator (Enslein et al., 1987b). The other eight were members of rarely occurring classes. There are actually four models, two for compounds with rings, and two for compounds without rings. For compounds without rings, one model predicts whether the compound will produce severe skin irritation, the other whether the irritation is likely to be mild/moderate. An identical scheme is used for the compounds containing rings.

The estimation then proceeds in two steps: first an SAR equation is used to determine whether the compound is likely to produce severe irritation; if it is not, then the second equation predicts whether the irritation is likely to be mild/moderate, or negative.

The performance of this estimator is shown in Table 4.

TABLE 4
Performance of Skin Irritation Estimator

Class	Submodel	Overall Accuracy	Indeterminates
Non-Ring	Severe vs. others	95%	12%
	Negative vs. others	95%	2%
Ring	Severe vs. others	91%	16%
	Negative/mild vs. mod./sev.	90%	16%
Global accuracy		93%	12%

Rabbit Eye Irritation. This estimator is similar to that for rabbit skin irritation, in that it consists of four separate models, two for compounds without rings and two for chemicals with rings (Enslein et al., in press). In this estimator the second ring model separates negatives and milds from moderates, rather than negatives from all others.

The data sources for these SAR models are, on the whole, the same as for the skin irritation models, except that very few data of those supplied by the U.S. Army could be used, inasmuch as this organization used much lower doses for the assay, and that no compounds were supplied by RIFM, as they do not routinely test fragrances for eye irritation. Just as for the skin irritation data, the results produced by Smyth et al. and Marhold had to be harmonized with the Draize scoring system.

The sources are given in Table 5, and the performance of this estimator is shown in Table 6.

Note the relatively high proportion of indeterminates, i.e., chemicals that could not be classified by the SAR models. We believe these reflect "noise" in the data, i.e., inaccuracies in classifying a compound as producing, for example, mild irritation when in fact it should have been called moderate.

A worked example of an eye irritation estimate will be found in Section III below.

Rat Oral LD50. This SAR estimator is based on compounds listed in the Registry of Toxic Effects of Chemical Substances (RTECS) (Lewis, 1984). RTECS lists only the

TABLE 5
Eye Irritation Model Data Sources

Source	Scoring Method	Number of Compounds
Smyth et al.	10-point	682
Marhold, Institute of Hygiene	10-point	313
Various Draize scores	Draize	63
Other	Various	104
		1,162

TABLE 6
Performance of Eye Irritation Estimator

Class	Submodel	Overall Accuracy	Indeterminates
Non-Ring	Severe vs. others	90%	31%
	Negative vs. mild/moderate	90%	15%
Ring	Severe vs. others	88%	24%
	Negative vs. mild/moderate	93%	29%
Global accuracy		91%	25%

lowest (i.e., most toxic) value found in the literature. Consequently, estimates derived from this model are worst-case estimates, and can easily differ from other rat oral LD50 assays for the same compound by a factor of ten (Hunter et al., 1978). This bias also has an effect on the best correlation that can be obtained with the predictive variables, inasmuch as the deviation in the LD50 value from the average for a compound that one would obtain were an assay to be repeated many times appears as noise.

The rat oral LD50 estimator (Enslein et al., 1983) is based on 2066 chemicals, covering a wide variety of structures. Certain classes, however, were excluded because of their perturbation of the model. These are compounds which include silicon, boron, arsenic, phosphorus, and all organometallics, as well as cholinesterase inhibitors.

The performance of this model is shown in Table 7.

It can be seen that almost 50% of the compounds are predicted within a factor of two, and essentially all within a factor of eight. This level of accuracy is comparable to that achieved by repeated performance of actual bioassays of the same substance in different laboratories.

AN EXAMPLE OF EYE IRRITATION ESTIMATION

In this Section, we will demonstrate the steps involved in making an eye irritation estimate for 4-Aminosalicylic acid (4-AA). The structure is shown in Fig. 1A.

TABLE 7
Rat Oral LD_{50} Model Performance

Factor	Percent of Compounds Predicted within the Factor
1.2	15
1.5	30
2.0	49
5.0	65
8.0	95

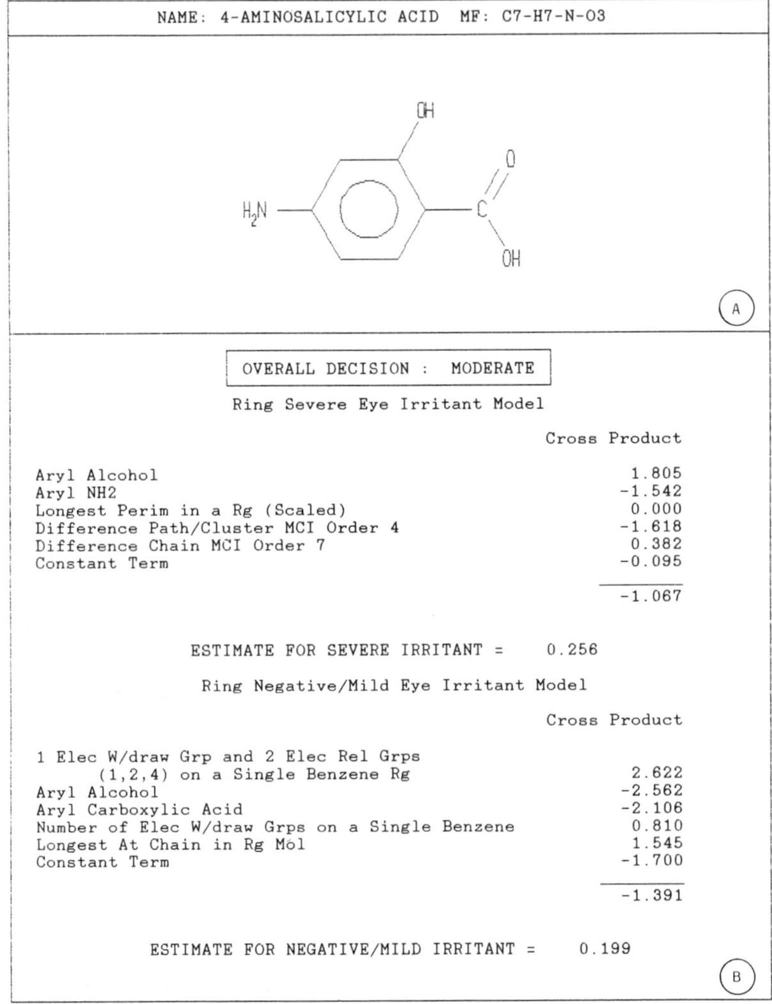

FIGURE 1A. Structure of compound for estimation.

FIGURE 1B. Calculation of eye irritation estimate.

Estimation. Fig. 1B shows the estimate itself. Since this compound contains a ring, the ring models are being used. The first model classifies the compound as to the probability that it is a severe eye irritant. Note that the probability is 0.256, indicating that there is only a low probability that its irritancy potential is severe. Figs. 2A-2E

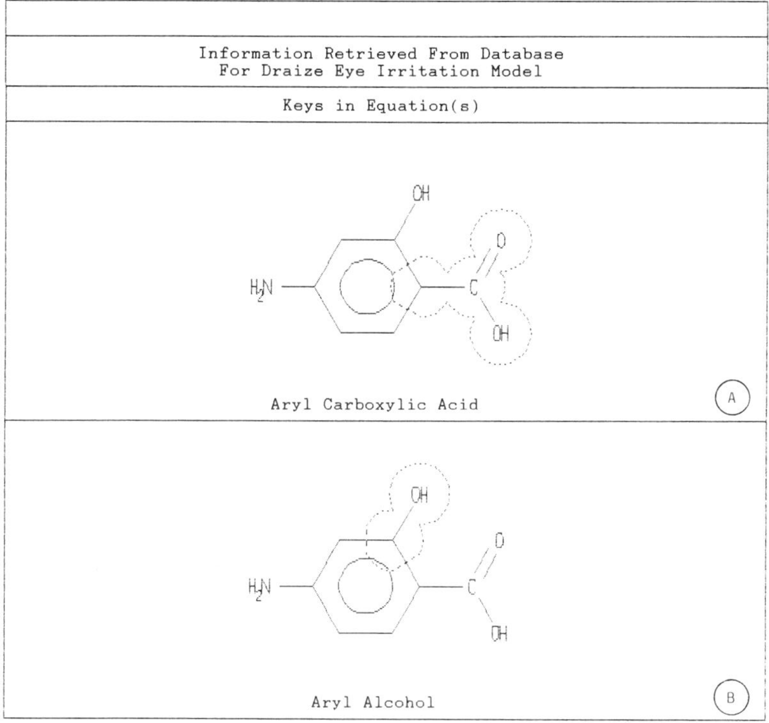

FIGURES 2A-2E. Substructures used in eye irritation estimate. Each substructure is encircled.

show the substructures that have been identified in the compound as being in the equations from which the estimate is being computed, as well as in 4-AA itself. Note that the entire structure is "covered" by substructures appearing in the equations.

Going back to Fig. 1B, the probability of severe irritation is calculated from the sum of cross-products. Each cross-product is calculated from the value of the corresponding parameter times that parameter's coefficient in the SAR equation. A positive cross-product increases the probability of severe irritancy, a negative cross-product reduces it.

The second equation shows that the probability for the compound being a negative or mild irritant is 0.199, i.e., low. Integrating the results from both equations then results in the Overall Decision that the eye irritation potential for 4-AA is Moderate. (Inasmuch as there are only three possible categories when negative and mild are combined, two equations are sufficient to arrive at a decision.)

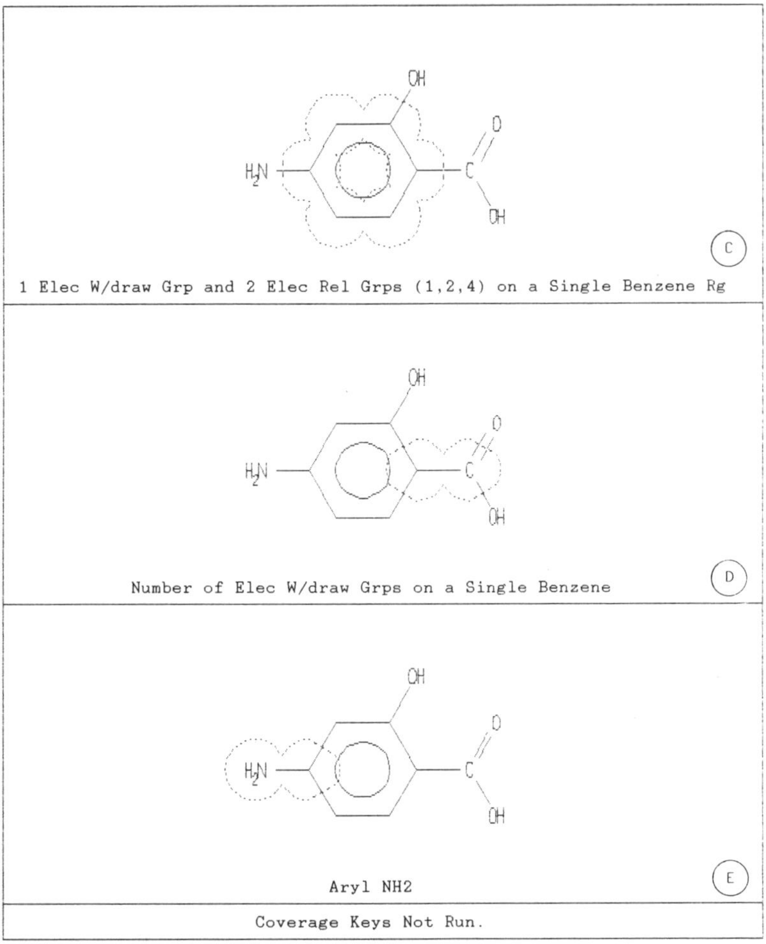

FIGURE 2. (Continued).

Note that it is possible to determine from the equations the parameters which have a substantial influence on the estimate. For example, for the "severe" model, the positive contribution of aryl alcohol is essentially balanced by the negative contribution of aryl amine. The deciding factor is then the topology of the compound, represented (in part) by the "Difference Path/ Cluster MCI (Molecular Connectivity Index) Order 4." This parameter represents the parts of 4-AA shown in Fig. 2F, and takes into account the valence, and therefore the types, of atoms in the structure. One

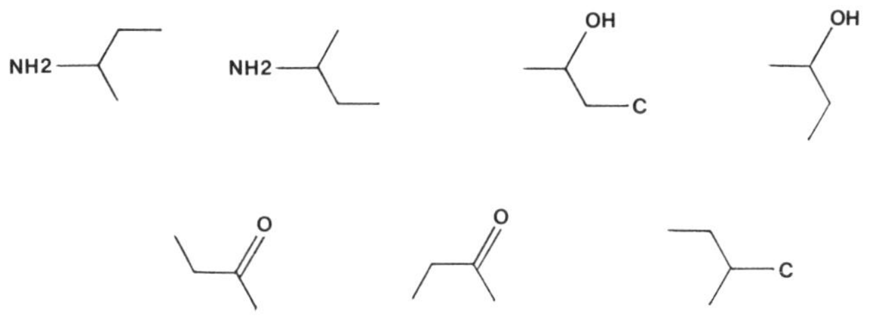

FIGURE 2F. Components of Difference Path/Cluster Molecular Connectivity Index Order 4 in 4-AA.

interpretation of this finding is that this substructure may match the receptor for eye irritation. It is thus possible, by careful analysis, to determine the influential factors in an estimate, and use this information as a guide in further investigations.

Validation. The TOPKAT program will always compute an estimate for a compound. The question is whether there is meaning in the estimate. To establish a confidence level for an estimate, it is useful to examine the compounds in the data base from which the SAR model was developed for the important substructures present in the compound to be estimated. Figs. 3A-3I show the structures found in the eye irritation data base with a search of aryl alcohol and amine. Fig. 3A, for example, shows the RTECS identifier (CB5470000), the CAS Number (116-84-7), the RTECS Code for the source of the data (28ZPAK-,83,72), the eye irritation severity (MILD), whether the compound was used in the model (Yes), and the name of the chemical. The first five compounds which were found contain the anthraquinone structure, and are too different from 4-AA to be considered for validation purposes. The last four, however, are reasonably similar. Note that three of the four produced moderate eye irritation; the fourth had a mild irritancy rating.

For the second equation, we have chosen to examine compounds with the aryl carbocyclic acid substituent, since this was an important negative parameter. These compounds are shown in Figs. 4A-4G. Of the seven compounds, three are mild, three moderate, and one severe. Of the milds, compounds 4E and 4G have two carbocyclic acid substituents, which reduce their irritation level below moderate. The only difference between the severe, salicylic acid, and the structure we are estimating is the amino group, which from the first equation is seen to reduce irritation severity. The preponderance of the evidence is such that the estimate for 4-Aminosalicylic acid can be given a high level of confidence. In fact, the bioassay for that compound results in moderate skin irritation.

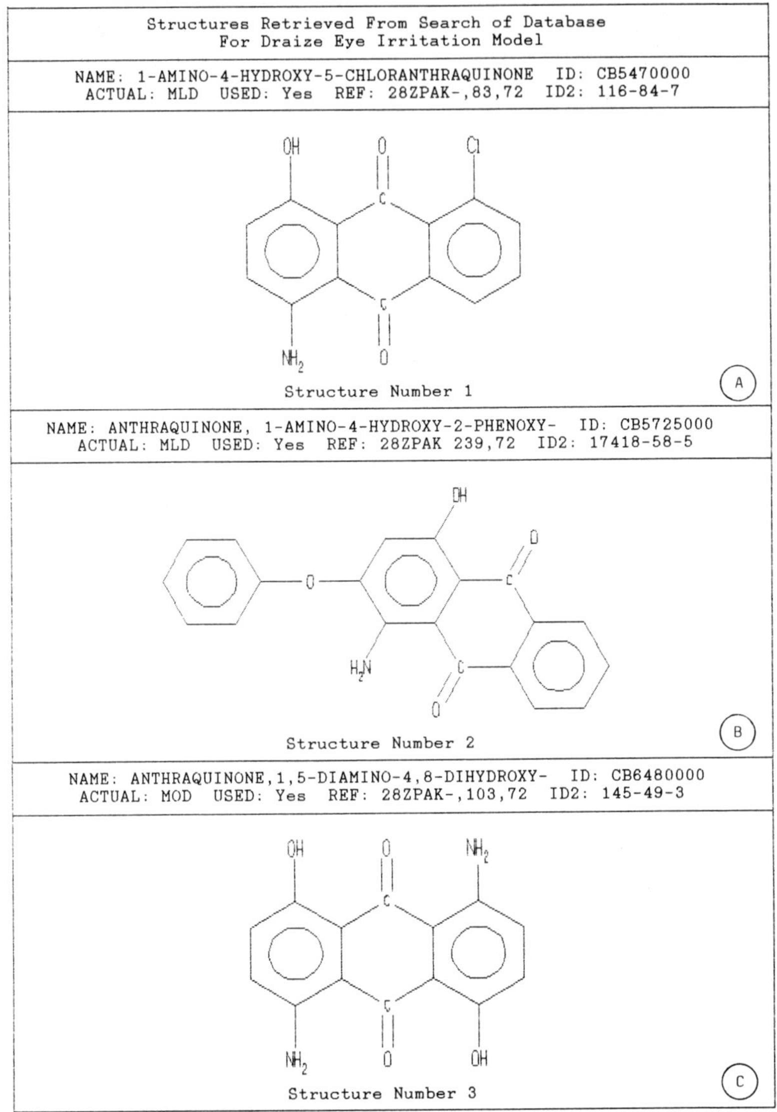

FIGURES 3A-3I. Structures used for validation of "severe" irritant estimate.

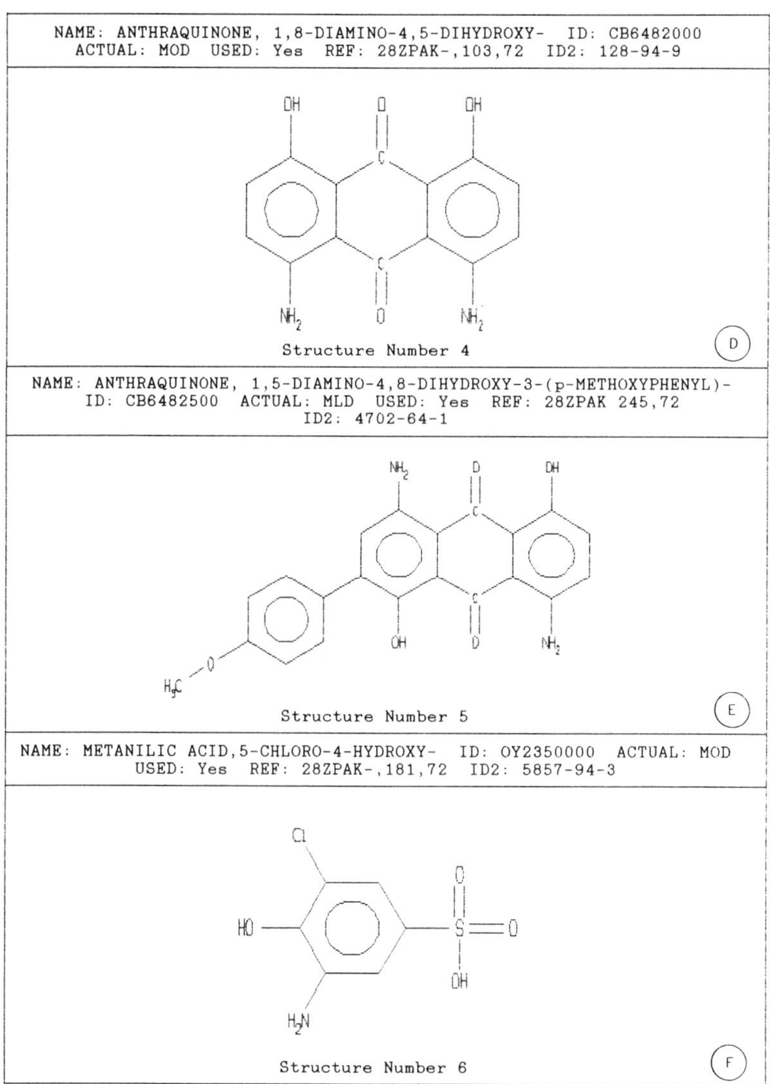

FIGURE 3. (Continued).

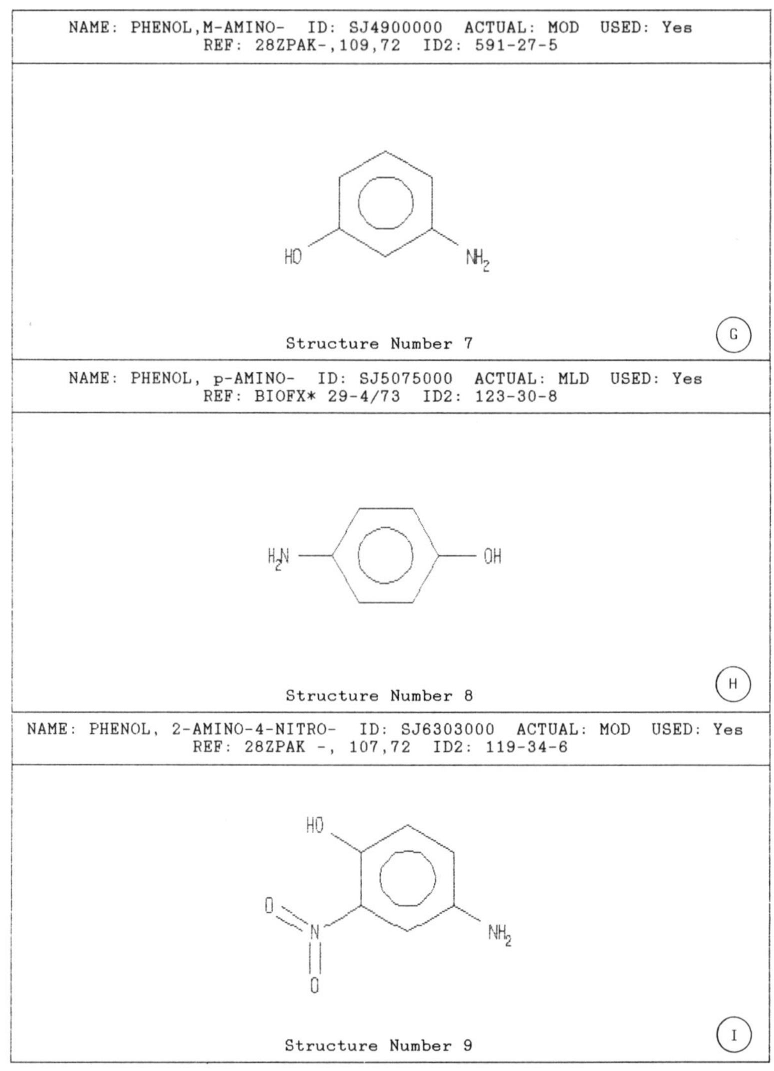

FIGURE 3. (Continued).

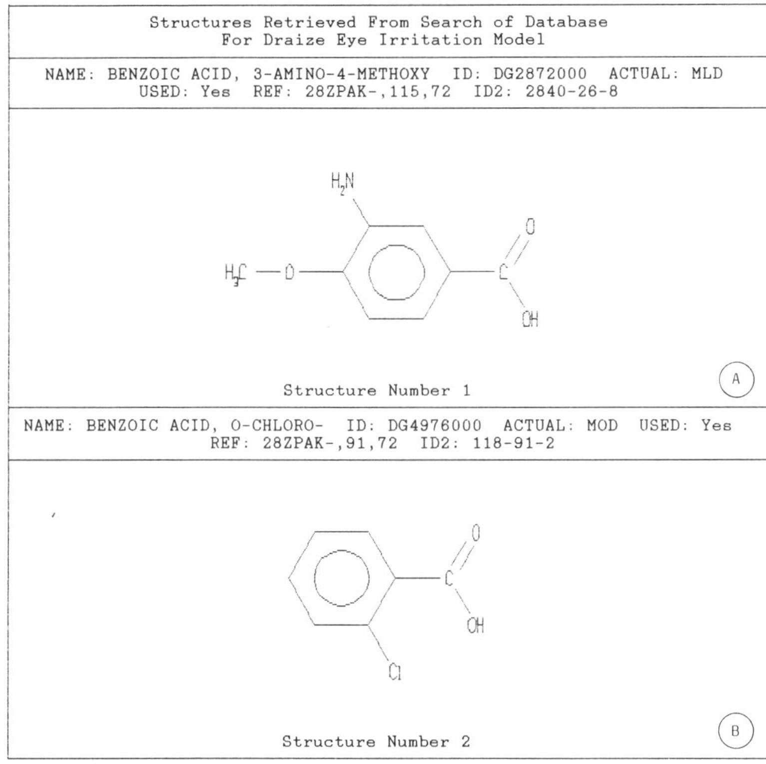

FIGURES 4A-4G. Structures used for validation of "negative/mild" irritation estimate.

DISCUSSION

We have described a system of SAR equations and their computer implementation useful for the estimation of toxic endpoints. These SAR models can be used in a variety of applications.

At the **chemical discovery** level, the potential toxic effects of a set of related compounds can be investigated before synthesis to select for further investigation those chemicals with the lesser probabilities of producing toxic effects, at considerable savings in research expenditure, since fewer compounds will need to be synthesized, and due to avoidance of blind alleys. The models can be used for test **prioritization**, such as selecting those chemicals in an environment which are most likely to have toxic effects for priority attention. SAR models can be used by **regulatory** agencies to

FIGURE 4. (Continued).

determine the possible toxic effects of chemicals for which data insufficient to render decisions have been submitted, and to gain insight into possible toxicity problems. SAR models can also be used to investigate possible **metabolites** and toxicity mechanisms, due to the ability of making computer-based **structural modifications** and observing the effects on the modelled toxic endpoints. **Hazard identification** is a natural outgrowth of several of the above applications, and is particularly cogent for the carcinogenicity model.

The SAR equations used in the TOPKAT program are, in many ways, very similar to those used for the estimation of physico-chemical parameters, such as the octanol/water partition coefficient (log P) (Leo and Weininger, 1984). In the estimation of log P, the effects of different components of a chemical are added; terms accounting for the interaction between components are also introduced. It should thus not come as a surprise that similar equations are effective for toxic endpoints.

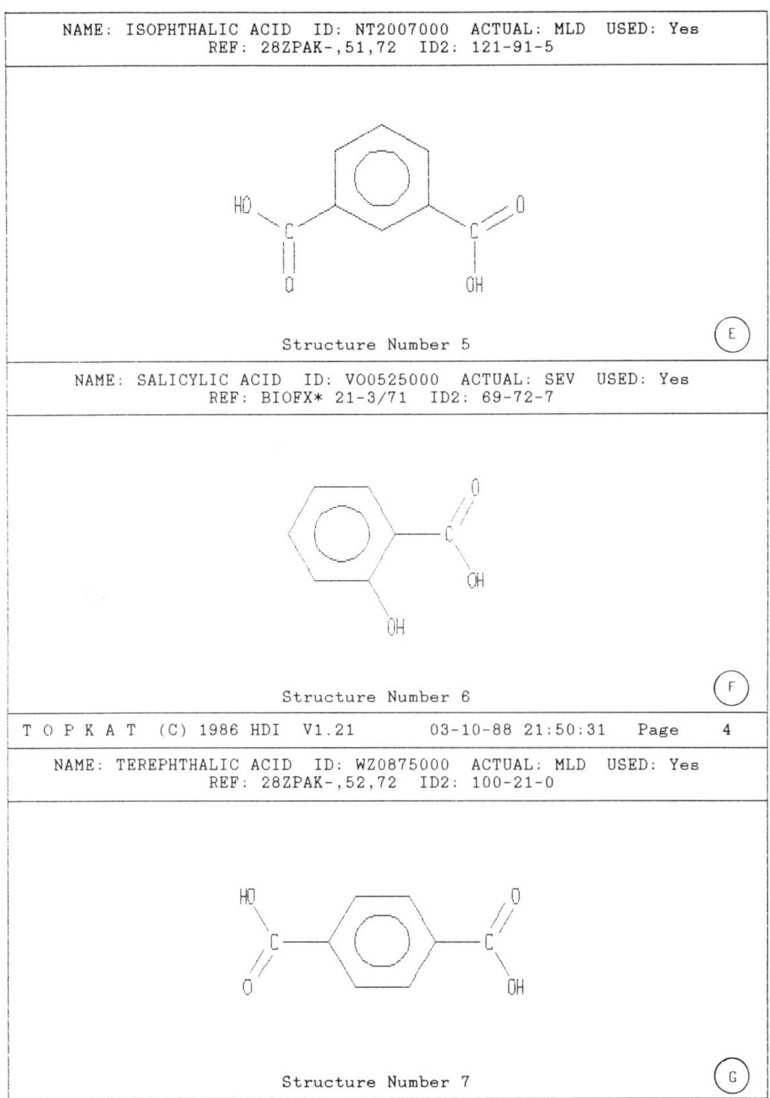

FIGURE 4. (Continued).

The TOPKAT program differs from the CASE system (Klopman, 1984) in three fundamental ways:

1. The TOPKAT program uses predetermined parameters for the modelling of the toxic endpoint, whereas CASE generates many atom-centered fragments for the particular example at hand. This difference has a profound effect on
2. The statistical methods used for modelling. Whereas CASE uses an essentially open-ended system developed for applications with a large objects-to-parameters ratio but applied to the converse situation, the TOPKAT program uses closed statistical methods, the effects of which can be verified through extensive diagnostics to arrive at robust equations; and
3. The TOPKAT program includes elaborate methodology for the validation of an estimate based on the chemicals that contributed to the estimate, whereas in the CASE system, one has to accept the toxicity estimate on the premise that only interpolation within, not extrapolation outside the chemical space used for modelling has been done.

This point needs reemphasis: both the TOPKAT program and the CASE system will produce estimates of toxic endpoints, but it is only after each estimate has been thoroughly validated that one can have any confidence in the prediction, notwithstanding the performance of either method on prior examples.

The chemical used for the example of Section III was completely "covered" by the substructures used in the calculation of its irritancy estimate. There frequently are chemicals which include features that are not used in the calculation of the estimate. In those instances, it is useful to examine the data base from which the model was developed to determine whether those features were represented in the data base. The fact that a particular feature was present with sufficient frequency and yet was not used in the estimate is an indication that it was not important enough to contribute to the explanation of the endpoint. Thus, one can feel confident that even though the feature was not used in the calculation of the estimate, its effect is nevertheless taken into account.

The current SAR models cannot handle mixtures if there is a presupposition of interaction between the components, i.e., synergism or antagonism, due to the fact that very few data exist for such mixtures. In cases of simple additivity of effects, the current SAR models are effective.

Thus, just as bioassays and *in vitro* methods have their limitations, so do SAR models. In addition to the points mentioned above, these include also the sometimes limited data base on which an SAR model is based, the temptation to extrapolate beyond the confines of the model, and the noise inherent in the bioassays on which the models are based. Within these constraints SAR models have a considerable potential in reducing the number of animals used in toxicity testing.

REFERENCES

CODE OF FEDERAL REGULATIONS, Food and Drugs, Vol. 21 (1979). Superintendent of Documents, Washington, DC 20402.

DRAIZE, J.H., WOODWARD, G. and CALVERY, H.O. (1944). Methods for study of irritation and toxicity of substances applied topically to the skin and mucous membranes. J. Pharmacol. Exp. Therap. **82**:377.

ENSLEIN, K., LANDER, T.R., TOMB, M.E. and CRAIG, P.N. (1983). A predictive model for estimating rat oral LD50 values. Benchmark Papers in Toxicology. Princeton Scientific Publishers, Princeton, New Jersey.

ENSLEIN, K. (1984). Estimation of toxicological endpoints by structure-activity relationships. Pharm. Rev. **36**:131S-135S.

ENSLEIN, K., BLAKE, B.W., TOMB, M.E. and BORGSTEDT, H.H. (1986/87). Prediction of Ames test results by structure-activity relationships. In Vitro Toxicol. **1**:33–44.

ENSLEIN, K., BORGSTEDT, H.H., TOMB, M.E., BLAKE, B.W. and HART, J.B. (1987a). A structure-activity prediction model of carcinogenicity based on NCI/NTP assays and food additives. Toxicol. Industr. Health **3**:267–287.

ENSLEIN, K., BORGSTEDT, H.H., BLAKE, B.W. and HART, J.B. (1987b). Prediction of rabbit skin irritation severity by structure-activity relationships. In Vitro Toxicol. **1**:129-147.

ENSLEIN, K., BLAKE, B.W., TUZZEO, T.M., BORGSTEDT, H.H. and HART, J.B. Estimation of rabbit eye irritation scores by structure-activity equations. (In press).

GRIESEMER, R.A. and CUETO, C. (1980). Toward a classification scheme for degrees of experimental evidence for the carcinogenicity of chemicals for animals. IARC Scientific Publications **27**:259–281.

HANSCH, C. and LEO, A. (1979). Substituent Constants for Correlation Analysis in Chemistry and Biology. Wiley, New York.

HUNTER, W.J., LINGK, W. and RECHT, P. (1978). An Intercomparison Study Conducted by the Commission of the European Communities on the Determination of the Single Administration of Toxicity in Rats. Commission of the European Communities, Health and Safety Directorate, Luxembourg.

KLOPMAN, G. (1984). Artificial intelligence approach to structure-activity studies. Computer-automated structure evaluation of biological activity of organic molecules. J. Amer. Chem. Soc. **106**:7315-7321.

LEO, A. and WEININGER, D. (1984). CLOGP3, Version 3.2. User Reference Manual. Medicinal Chemistry Project, Pomona College, Claremont, CA.

LEWIS, R.J. Sr. (1984). Registry of Toxic Effects of Chemical Substances. DHHS, Cincinnati, OH 45226.

MARHOLD, J.V. (1972). J. Results Toxicological Test Substances and Preparations. Prague, Czechoslovakia.

OPDYKE, D.L.J. and LETIZIA, C. (1982-83). Monographs on fragrance raw materials. Fd. Chem. Tox. **21**:645–667 (1983), 833–875 (1983), 20 Suppl (1982).

SMYTH, H.F. and CARPENTER, C.P. (1944). The place of the range finding test in the industrial toxicology laboratory. J. Ind. Hyg. Toxicol. **26**:269–273.

SMYTH, H.F. and CARPENTER, C.P. (1948). Further experience with the range finding test in the industrial toxicology laboratory. J. Ind. Hyg. Toxicol. **30**:63–68.

SMYTH, H.F., CARPENTER, C.P. and WEIL, C.S. (1949). Range finding toxicity data, list III. J. Ind. Hyg. Toxicol. **31**:60–62.

SMYTH, H.F., CARPENTER, C.P. and WEIL, C.S. (1951). Range finding toxicity data, list IV. AMA Arch. Ind. Hyg. **4**:119–122.

SMYTH, H.F., CARPENTER, C.P., WEIL, C.S. and POZZANI, V.C. (1954). Range finding toxicity data, list V. AMA Arch. Ind. Hyg. **10**:61–68.

SMYTH, H.F., CARPENTER, C.P., WEIL, C.S., POZZANI, V.C. and STRIEGEL, J.A. (1962). Range finding toxicity data: list VI. Am. Ind. Hyg. Assoc. J. **23**:95–107.

SNAPINN, S.M. and KNOKE, J.D. (1985). An evaluation of smoothed classification error rate estimators. Technometrics **27**:199–206.

U.S. DEPARTMENT OF HEALTH AND HUMAN SERVICES (1985). Fourth Annual Report on Carcinogens. NTP Publication 85–002.

WEIL, C.S. and SCALA, R.A. (1971). Study of intra- and inter-laboratory variability in the results of rabbit eye and skin irritation tests. Toxicol. Appl. Pharmacol. **19**:276–360.

Received February 26, 1988
Accepted March 30, 1988

IN VITRO TECHNIQUES IN TERATOLOGY

GEORGE P. DASTON AND ROBERT A. D'AMATO

**Human and Environmental Safety Division
Miami Valley Laboratories
The Procter & Gamble Company
Cincinnati, Ohio**

INTRODUCTION

Considerable effort has gone into the development of alternative methods for the assessment of developmental toxicity. The principal impetus for the development of these assays is the need for more rapid, cost effective and less animal intensive means of obtaining at least some data on the developmentally toxic potential of new chemicals. The traditional methods for assessing developmental toxicity, specifically the Segment 2 study or some variation of it, have proven to be relatively reliable in predicting human teratogenic hazards; however, these protocols are labor intensive, time consuming and costly. The capacity of the typical industrial laboratory to conduct these assessments is far outstripped by the capacity of synthetic chemists to create new chemical entities. As a result, developmental toxicity testing has not kept up with the appearance of new chemicals in commerce. The magnitude of the deficit is enormous. There are approximately 60,000 chemicals currently in commercial or industrial use, but developmental toxicity data are available for only about 3000. Thousands of newly synthesized organic chemicals are registered with the American Chemical Society each month, and there are already more than six million on file. Thus, there is a continually expanding need for rapid and inexpensive screening techniques to provide information on the potential of chemicals to adversely affect development.

A number of *in vitro* test methods have been developed to assess the potential of chemicals to cause developmental toxicity. These include assays using established cell lines which evaluate a single, developmentally relevant endpoint of toxicity; primary cultures derived from embryos which assess one or more developmental processes; cultures of organ primordia derived from embryos; or intact embryos, including both rodent embryos in culture and free living embryos of sub-mammalian species. Although free living embryos are not truly *in vitro* preparations, they have been used as the basis for rapid teratogenicity assays, and will be discussed.

---

1. Address correspondence to: Dr. George P. Daston, Miami Valley Laboratories, The Procter & Gamble Company, P.O. Box 398707, Cincinnati, OH 45239.
2. Key words: alternative methods, developmental toxicity, teratology.

This review will describe: 1) *in vitro* developmental toxicity screens which are available, including their state of development and validation; 2) the potential applications of *in vitro* developmental toxicity screens in industrial, regulatory and basic research settings; 3) the philosophy behind the development of screens to assess abnormal development; and 4) the interpretation of data from *in vitro* screens.

It should be noted that developmental toxicity has four manifestations: teratogenicity, embryo/fetal death, growth retardation and functional deficit. Most *in vitro* screens have been designed to detect agents which cause terata. The bulk of the developmental toxicology literature indicates that teratogens can also cause the other manifestations of developmental toxicity; however, there are sufficient reports in the literature of materials which are embryolethal and/or growth retarding, but not teratogenic. This may be a reflection that the commonly used *in vivo* methods are biased towards producing this type of developmental toxicity (Johnson and Christian, 1984), but that the mechanisms which produce these types of developmental toxicity are the same as those which produce terata. Alternatively, these phenomena may be produced by different mechanisms. If the latter is true, then *in vitro* screens designed to detect teratogens may not be sensitive to all developmental toxicants. It is not within the scope of this review to answer this question, but keep in mind that most of the *in vitro* screens discussed are presented as *teratogen* screens, which may or may not be equivalent to *developmental toxicant* screens.

POTENTIAL USES FOR *IN VITRO* DEVELOPMENTAL TOXICITY ASSAYS

In vitro methods have been used for decades to study normal developmental processes, and have been more recently applied to the study of abnormal development. The purpose of using *in vitro* methods to study mechanisms is, of course, to simplify the experimental system sufficiently that the effects of a test chemical on specific biological processes may be evaluated. For example, cellular assays which model processes important to development may be used to study the effects of teratogens on those processes.

Intact rodent embryo culture also has been used in basic research on teratogenic mechanisms. This assay has utility in eliminating maternal factors such as compound delivery and metabolism, as well as maternal stress or disease states which might confound interpretation of results. One of the most effective uses of rodent embryo culture is in determining whether the parent compound or a metabolite is teratogenic. Since the embryo has little xenobiotic metabolizing capability, individual metabolites may be added to the culture to determine whether they have any toxicity. As an example, rodent embryo culture has been used to demonstrate that cyclophosphamide requires metabolism to be teratogenic (Fantel et al., 1979; Hales, 1981), and that only one or two of the metabolites of cyclophosphamide are teratogenic. In a related use, mouse embryo culture has been used to investigate the factors responsible for the developmental toxicity associated with maternal diabetes by adding single abnormal serum factors (e.g. excess insulin, glucose, ketone bodies, etc.) to the cultures (Sadler et al., 1985).

There are many other excellent examples of the use of *in vitro* methods to study teratogenic mechanisms, but the main purpose of this review is to evaluate the use of these methods as screening tools. At present, none of the *in vitro* assays has been sufficiently validated, or been sufficiently predictive, to gain wide acceptance as an all purpose screen for developmental toxicants. However, it is important to note that many assays could be used now for specific applications, especially in industrial product development. It is now common for industrial synthetic chemists to create families of related chemicals in the initial stage of product development to increase the likelihood of finding the congener with the most desirable qualities, and preferably with the least toxicity. Rapid *in vitro* screens could be used to rank order the teratogenic potential of chemical families so that the ones with the least toxicity could be further developed. Since closely related chemicals would presumably act via a common teratogenic mechanism, then a single *in vitro* screen, if sensitive to this mechanism, could be used to judge the relative potencies of all members of the family. Kistler (1987) has used an *in vitro* mouse limb bud cell screen to successfully rank the teratogenic potential of a large series of synthetic retinoids. *In vitro* methods are also advantageous in these circumstances because new materials are typically synthesized in small quantities—too small to characterize teratogenic potential *in vitro*, but usually sufficient for *in vitro* assays. Determining teratogenic potential at an early stage of product development would be a significant factor in the decision to synthesize larger quantities of a new material.

Alternative methods are also of interest for governmental regulatory bodies as a means of setting the order in which they ask for more comprehensive testing of chemicals for developmental toxicity. This is a considerably different application from the one described above, as these chemicals would probably not be closely related and may act through a variety of teratogenic mechanisms. An extreme example of this would be the testing of complex mixtures of unknown chemical composition derived from hazardous waste sites as a means of prioritizing those sites for cleanup. Such an application would require a very versatile screen which is not only sensitive to a variety of teratogenic mechanisms, but is also capable of testing chemicals with a variety of physical chemical properties.

An additional reason for pursuing alternative test methods is the potential ethical concern raised by a segment of the society over the use of laboratory animals in safety testing. Many of the alternative test systems use established cell lines, and therefore largely eliminate the use of animals. Others rely on intact non-mammalian embryos, systems which do not require the sacrifice of mammals, but do use relatively large numbers of lower vertebrates and invertebrates. Still others use cells or organs derived from living embryos, or the embryos themselves, although all of these are more economical than standard reproductive toxicity tests. It is an obligation and a goal for all toxicologists to reduce the number of animals which they use whenever possible; however, it is an even greater obligation to carry out all the research necessary to ensure that the public health is protected. Therefore, consideration of animal use is important, but it must be approached with assurances for protection of human safety.

As for reduction in animal use, the standard Segment 2 developmental toxicity assay typically requires 100 laboratory mammals; 25 animals in each of four doses groups (including a control). Alternative test methods would use fewer lab mammals. Procedures using primary cultures of embryos, or intact rodent embryos, generally require only 10% of the number of animals as standard *in vitro* procedures. Other tests using established cell lines require no additional use of lab animals. Assay systems using intact sub-mammalian embryos obviously use no laboratory mammals; however, they do employ comparable numbers of embryos as the standard procedures.

In this review we will consider the attributes which an alternative test must possess in order to be useful for screening purposes as well as the problems of developing such a screen and the ways in which methods development has been approached. The types of *in vitro* assays which are now available will be reviewed. These include *in vitro* tests with mammalian embryos and free living non-mammalian embryos; and *in vitro* tests using established cell lines, primary cultures of embryonal cells or organs. The application of quantitative data from *in vitro* assays in risk assessment will be discussed.

DESIRABLE ATTRIBUTES OF AN *IN VITRO* TERATOGEN SCREEN

There are two essential attributes which any alternative system must possess in order to be useful as a screen: first, it must be predictive of toxicity in humans; second, it must be quantitative, having graded responses to increasing concentrations of the toxicant (in other words, it must generate dose-response relationships). In addition to these, there are several other attributes which are highly desirable and may greatly enhance the versatility and utility of a screen. Similar criteria were arrived at by the Consensus Workshop on In Vitro Teratogenesis Testing sponsored by U.S. regulatory agencies in 1981 (Kimmel et al., 1982).

Prediction of Human Teratogenicity. The first essential attribute—prediction of teratogenic potential in humans—is intuitively obvious. However, for several reasons demonstration of predictiveness to man must be indirect, through comparisons to laboratory animal studies. First, there are only a limited number of known human teratogens, about twenty. This is probably too few substances against which to compare the predictiveness of any screen. Second, the dose levels required to cause developmental toxicity in humans are not firmly established, except for certain pharmaceutical agents; thus, it may be possible to make only qualitative comparisons between human data and that generated by an alternative system. Quantitative assessments of the predictiveness of the test (i.e., that it correctly classifies developmental toxicants at concentrations which are relevant to *in vivo* dose levels) can only be made through comparisons to developmental toxicity data generated in controlled animal experiments.

Accuracy has two components: a predictive screen must not only detect developmental toxicants, but it also must distinguish these from non-toxicants. In other words, it must be sensitive and specific. A sensitive test is one which successfully identifies developmental toxicants, with few false negatives. A specific test successfully classifies non-toxicants, with few false positives. A successful test would generate very few false positives or negatives.

The equivalent importance of sensitivity and specificity should be taken into account in the design of protocols to validate alternative tests. In order to document that a screen has both characteristics, a similar number of known developmental toxicants and non-toxicants must be tested. The known developmental toxicants tested should be representative of known teratogenic mechanisms, represent a wide range of potencies, and have various physical chemical properties. The non-toxicants should represent the same broad range of physical chemical properties, and it is preferable that some of these are structurally similar to known developmental toxicants.

As with any test method, some level of error is to be expected and must be taken into account in interpreting the results. Interpretation would be facilitated if all of the errors are either false negatives or false positives. If all errors were false negatives, then any negative in the *in vitro* assay would be further tested in a more meaningful traditional *in vivo* assay. This would be useful when the alternative is used as a preliminary screen during product development, to eliminate potent teratogens from further development or testing. On the other hand, a test method which generates few false negatives but more false positive results may be more acceptable if the developmental toxicity of a substance will be evaluated solely by the *in vitro* screen. In such instances, errors would be on the side of caution. No toxicants would escape notice, but a number of non-toxic substances would be mistakenly classified as being potentially teratogenic.

It may be possible to minimize either false negatives or false positives (but not both) by manipulating the upper concentration limit of chemicals used in the test. The U.S. National Toxicology Program (NTP) reported the accuracy of two *in vitro* teratogen screens in detecting the developmental toxicity of 44 substances as a function of maximum concentration used in the data analysis (NTP, 1986; Steele et al., 1987). They used concentrations ranging from 0.05 mM to 40 mM. As might be expected, more false negatives were generated when data from only the lowest concentrations were evaluated. For example, at a concentration level of 0.05 mM, all the non-teratogens were correctly classified, giving an overall accuracy of 54.2%. As concentration was increased, the number of false negatives decreased and the number of false positives increased. Overall accuracy was highest at chemical concentrations of 10-20 mM, when it was 70.8%. At higher concentrations accuracy was lower and the number of false positives became extremely high: 87.5%. Thus, manipulation of concentrations has its limits: the overall accuracy of the test battery decreased sharply at concentrations which optimized either false negatives or false positives.

Concentration-Response Relationships. The second required attribute for an *in vitro* developmental toxicity screen is that it be able to demonstrate concentration-response relationships. Developmental toxicity is a concentration-dependent phenomenon. It has a threshold and the severity of effect increases with increasing concentration of toxicant. As the example for the NTP *in vitro* study demonstrates, the classification of a substance as teratogenic or non-teratogenic depended on the concentration used. Thus, it is inappropriate to label a material as teratogenic or non-teratogenic without also providing information about dosage. Any screen for developmental toxicity, *in vivo* or *in vitro*, must be capable of indicating a no observable effect level (NOEL), a lowest observable effect level (LOEL), and concentration-response curves in order to be of use in predicting teratogenic potential.

Other Desirable Attributes. A third important attribute for an *in vitro* screen is that it must be able to accommodate substances of varying physical and chemical properties. These may include differences in physical state (gases vs. liquids or solutions), water solubility, light sensitivity, etc.

Most of the *in vitro* test methods, and tests using free living aquatic embryos, are limited in their ability to accommodate hydrophobic compounds, although there have been some procedures published which may be useful in solving this problem. The obvious solution is to use an amphiphilic solvent system, but many of these are teratogenic (e.g. ethanol), or may be limited in their ability to retain a hydrophobic material in an aqueous solution. Kitchin and Ebron (1984) tested a variety of amphiphilic solvent systems for their toxicity to explanted rat embryos, including DMSO, ethanol and acetone, and found that only an emulsion of corn oil and rat serum was completely non-toxic to embryos. Researchers using aquatic free living embryos have mixed hydrophobic compounds with solid vegetable shortening, and added this mixture to aquaria (T. Sabourin, personal communication). The test material slowly reaches equilibrium with the water, where it interacts with the embryos. Unfortunately, the actual dose to the embryo can not be estimated, and the maximum concentration of tests substance which can be achieved in the water must be very low.

Another useful characteristic for an *in vitro* screen is the ability to metabolize xenobiotics, or to be compatible with an exogenous metabolizing system which produces a spectrum of metabolites comparable to that which the human embryo would encounter. Metabolizing systems of varying complexity have been added to *in vitro* teratogen screens. The most common is the post-mitochondrial fraction (S-9) from a male rat liver homogenate, typically obtained after treatment with a monooxygenase system inducer (e.g. Aroclor) (Kitchin et al., 1981; Shepard et al., 1983; others).

Hepatic S-9 from other species has also been added to *in vitro* teratogen screens, such as male mouse S-9 to rat and mouse embryo culture (Daston et al., 1987). Another approach has been to add intact hepatocytes to *in vitro* cultures. This has been tried with some success with rat hepatocytes (Oglesby et al., 1986) and rat or human hepatoma cells (Brown and Kram, 1982) added to rat embryo cultures.

At least some *in vitro* systems have innate metabolic capabilities. Brown et al. (1986) have demonstrated xenobiotic metabolizing ability in mouse embryo limb bud and CNS cell culture, and there is some evidence that rat embryos *in utero* can metabolize polycyclic aromatic hydrocarbons (Shum et al., 1979). This activity is low compared with that of adult liver, but it is sufficient to detect at least some teratogens which require metabolic activation.

Another highly desirable quality in an alternative screen is that it have objective endpoints. This is almost obligatory if the test is to generate concentration-response curves, or be used in quantitative risk assessment. Examples of objective and continuous endpoints are the measurement of protein or DNA content, or embryo length, as indices of growth. Examples of discrete endpoints are death vs. survival, growth vs. no growth, etc.

APPROACHES TO *IN VITRO* SCREEN METHODS DEVELOPMENT

The purpose of *in vitro* methods development is to faithfully reproduce the biological phenomenon of interest in a simpler system than the intact animal. In the case of teratogen screens, the phenomenon of interest is embryonic development, and how it is affected by chemical insult. Unfortunately for the *in vitro* teratologist, embryonic development is perhaps the most complicated of all biological processes, and there are a number of ways in which teratogens can alter development. Wilson (1973) listed the general mechanisms by which teratogens may alter normal development (Table 1). A glance at the list is sufficient to ascertain that teratogens can act on chromosomes, by causing aberrations leading to large deletions or aneuploidy; on genes, by altering the expression of gene products (altering differentiation); on enzymes of intermediary metabolism; on cell membranes, by altering the way in which cells interact with each other or their environment. Osmotic imbalances are produced by affecting the systemic osmoregulatory physiology of the embryo. (Nutritional deficiencies are not a significant consideration in chemical teratogenesis). In order for an *in vitro* assay to be broadly applicable to screening, it must be able to detect teratogens acting by most or all of these mechanisms. Thus, a successful *in vitro* teratogen screen must be complex enough to model a number of developmental processes.

All of the cellular processes which are fundamental to development can take place *in vitro*. These include cell surface phenomena such as cell-cell recognition, adhesion, and gap junctional communication; cellular growth and division; and selective gene activity leading to the expression of a differentiated phenotype. It is also possible for

TABLE 1
Teratogenic Mechanisms[a]

1. Mutation
2. Chromosomal breaks or nondisjunction
3. Mitotic interference
4. Altered nucleic acid integrity or function
5. Lack of precursors, substrates, etc.
6. Altered energy sources
7. Enzyme inhibition
8. Fluid-osmolyte imbalance
9. Changed membrane characteristics

[a] From Wilson (1973).

higher order processes of development to occur in some *in vitro* preparations, including induction of differentiation by interaction with heterotypic cells; migration; and pattern formation.

There are a number of different strategies for developing *in vitro* teratogen screens. The first generation screens are simple systems which model a single developmentally relevant endpoint (e.g. cell adhesive properties, cell division) in an established cell line. These screens are rapid and cost effective, and are probably the easiest to carry out. However, they are not comprehensive screens since they only model a single developmental process. Only teratogens which affect that process will be detected in the assay.

It would be expected *a priori* that the accuracy of these tests in predicting teratogenicity would not be very good. This expectation was borne out in the only blind study conducted in two independent laboratories with two of these tests (NTP, 1986). Interestingly, one test, which measured cell division, was substantially more predictive of teratogenic potential than the other test, which measured cell adhesiveness. It is tempting to speculate from these results that teratogens which decrease cell division are much more prevalent than those which affect cell adhesiveness, and that cell division is a more important endpoint to include in a screen than is adhesiveness. It is more likely, however, that the teratogens used in this study (the list prepared by Smith et al., 1983) were biased towards those known to inhibit cell division. Thus, no conclusions on the relative prevalence of teratogenic mechanisms can be drawn.

It may be possible to improve the accuracy of single endpoint tests by combining a number of them as a battery. This was a consideration of the NTP when they conducted their validation study with two single endpoint tests. Interestingly, the accuracy of the battery was not greater than the accuracy of the better of the two tests (NTP, 1986). This indicates that such a battery may need more than two tests, or that selection of tests for inclusion in a battery must be done carefully. Of course, it is considerably more costly to run a battery of tests, and the problems of false positives becomes compounded, since a positive in any of the components of the battery would label the test agent as a potential teratogen.

An alternative strategy has been to develop more complicated assays in which a number of developmental processes occur. These systems are primary cultures of cells derived from embryonal tissues, or intact organ primordia from embryos. The cultures are typically composed of a number of different cell types, and presumably a number of different developmental events take place in the culture. These include growth and cell division, cell-cell interactions, and differentiation. It is anticipated that these tests will be more comprehensively predictive of teratogenicity than the single endpoint tests, and this is supported by data from the laboratories of the developers of the screens (see below for descriptions and accuracy rates of individual tests). However, none of these tests has been run through a rigorous testing program in an independent laboratory, so it is not possible to definitively conclude that these tests are more predictive.

A third strategy has been to use intact embryos as teratogen screens. Obviously, these undergo all of the fundamental processes of development, and physical relationships between tissue types is maintained so that it is certain that cell migration, pattern formation and morphogenetic movements can proceed normally. These must be considered to be the most comprehensive of the teratogen screens. On the other hand, much of the simplicity of *in vitro* systems is lost. Intact embryos *in vitro* are as complicated a system as embryos *in utero*, so there is little opportunity to learn anything about mechanism of action of a test agent. Although this is not the purpose of a screen, it may be useful information. There are complicating factors such as extra-embryonic membranes and large volumes of yolk or other extra-embryonic material which may not be comparable to those of the mammalian embryo, and which may influence the interaction of test material with the embryo; there tends to be a greater phylogenetic distance between these systems and humans than many of the other *in vitro* systems (although it is not clear whether this is significant in teratogen screening); and it is not yet possible to incorporate a xenobiotic metabolizing system which is relevant to humans into the media of non-mammalian embryos.

SUMMARY OF *IN VITRO* TERATOGEN SCREENS

Established Cell Lines. Assays using established cell lines measure a single endpoint which has some relevance to developmental processes at a cellular level, such as growth, cellular adhesion properties, cell-cell communication via gap junctions, and gene expression. These assays are attractive in that they are very quick and easy to execute, they require only small amounts of test substance, and they use no animals, as the cell lines are already established. On the other hand, because they are so simple, they are not comprehensive screens for developmental toxicity. Thus, they probably must be used in a battery, and even then may not be highly predictive.

TABLE 2
Summary of *In Vitro* Teratogen Screens[a]

Test Name	Test System	Endpoint(s)	Developmental Relevance	Reported Accuracy[b] (# of Materials Tested)	References
A. Established Cell Lines					
1. MOT	mouse ovarian tumor cells	attachment to lectin-coated surface	cell adhesiveness	72-79% (178)	Braun et al. 1982; Braun & Horowicz, 1983; NTP, 1986
2. HEPM	human embryonic palatal mesenchyme cells	cell growth (% of control)	cell proliferation	64-72% (99)	Pratt & Willis, 1985; NTP, 1986
3. Poxvirus proliferation	virus infected mammalian cells	formation of plaques by the poxvirus	expression of viral genome	86% (51)	Keller & Smith, 1982
4. Neuroblastoma cell differentiation	mouse neuroblastoma cells	differentiation of cells into neurons	cellular differentiation	86% (57)	Mummery et al., 1983
B. Primary Cultures of Embryonic Cells					
1. Chick embryo neural tube & limb bud	chick embryo cells from neural tube and limb buds	histological differentiation, synthesis of proteoglycans	cellular differentiation	93% (14)	Wilk et al., 1980; Greenberg et al., 1982
2. Mouse Limb Bud	mouse embryo limb bud cells	histological differentiation, synthesis of proteoglycans, DNA synthesis	cellular differentiation cell proliferation	89% (27)	Guntakatta et al., 1984; Kistler, 1987
3. Drosophila neuroblasts and myoblasts	neuroblasts and myoblasts from Drosophila embryos	histological differentiation	cellular differentiation	94% (100)	Bournias-Vardiabasis et al., 1983
4. Rat embryo micromass	Micromass cultures of rat embryo neural tube and limb bud cells	histological differentiation, synthesis of proteoglycans	cellular differentiation	91% (46)	Flint & Orton, 1984
5. Chick embryo neural retina cell culture	aggregate cultures of check embryo neural retina cells	formation of aggregates, growth, histological and biochemical differentiation	cell-cell interactions, cell proliferation, cellular differentiation	94% (17)	Daston et al., 1988

Test Name	Test System	Endpoint(s)	Developmental Relevance	Reported Accuracy[b] (# Materials Tested)	References
C. Intact Embryos					
1. Rat	post-implantation embryo culture	malformation, death growth retardation	assessment of development in an intact embryo	97% (38)	Schmid, 1985
2. CHEST	chick embryos (hen's egg)	malformation, death, growth retardation	assessment of development in an intact embryo	—(130)[c]	Jelinek, 1982; Jelinek et al., 1985
3. FETAX	frog embryos (*Xenopus laevis*)	malformation, death, growth retardation	assessment of development in an intact embryo	93% (43)	Dumont et al., 1983; Sabourin et al., 1985
4. Drosophila	fruit fly larvae	malformation, death growth retardation	assessment of development in an intact developing system	100% (8)	Schuler, 1982; Schuler et al. 1985; Ranganathan et al., 1987
5. Hydra	dissociated adult Hydra cells aggregated into a pellet	formation of an adult morph	assessment of reorganization and differentiation of cells	100% (24)[d]	Johnson and Gabel, 1983; Johnson et al., 1984

[a] Only assays which have undergone a validation program for teratogen screening are included.

[b] Accuracy is based on qualitative comparisons to the *in vitro* mammalian literature. Since developmental toxicity is a quantitative phenomenon, these accuracy values may be of little or no use in determining the predictiveness of a screen. (See text for a more detailed explanation).

[c] Comparisons to mammalian data were not made, so accuracy was not calculated by these authors.

[d] These data are expressed as A/D ratios and compared to A/D ratios from the mammalian developmental toxicology literature (see the text for a detailed description of A/D).

Since these assays are so rapid, a large number of chemicals has been screened in many of these. In the discussion below, we report the accuracy of these tests, which is a measure of the percentage of chemicals correctly classified as teratogens or non-teratogens. However, the reader should be aware that classification of materials as teratogenic or non-teratogenic without reference to concentration (dosage) may be misleading. For purposes of this review, we will report the accuracy rates which have been reported in the literature. These have been calculated by qualitatively comparing *in vitro* results to *in vivo* data from the literature. A positive response at any concentration in the *in vitro* test is considered to be an accurate response if there are any reports of developmental toxicity *in vivo* at any dosage. Obviously, such comparisons may not be of great use and are biased by the amount of published information on the *in vivo* developmental toxicity of each chemical.

MOT Assay. The MOT assay measures the attachment of ascitic mouse ovarian tumor cells (MOT cells) to a lectin (concanavalin A)-coated surface. Cellular adhesiveness is a generic property of embryonal cells; therefore, it is assumed that inhibition of adhesiveness by a chemical indicates teratogenic potential. The test chemical is added to a suspension of MOT cells which had been exposed to radiolabelled thymidine, and a plastic sheet coated with concanavalin A is placed in the culture vessel. Over a period of hours, the MOT cells normally adhere to the lectin-coated surface. Inhibition of this phenomenon by teratogens can be assessed by counting the radioactivity associated with the plastic sheets and comparing with control values (Braun et al., 1982).

This assay has been used to screen well over 100 substances, including known teratogens and non-teratogens (Braun et al., 1979; Braun et al., 1982; Braun and Horowicz, 1983; NTP, 1986; Steele et al., 1987). Rodent liver S-9 has successfully been used as a metabolic activating system for the MOT assay. The developer of the test reported an overall 79% accuracy as compared to *in vivo* results (Braun et al., 1979; Braun et al., 1982; Braun and Horowicz, 1983). The NTP used the MOT test along with the HEPM test (vide infra) as a battery, and reported a 72% agreement with *in vivo* results for the battery (NTP, 1986; Steele et al., 1987).

HEPM Assay. The HEPM assay measures the growth and proliferation of cells in the presence of test agents. Growth and division of cells is a fundamental process in developing tissues, and inhibition of this would be indicative of developmental toxicity. The cells used were originally derived from human embryonic palatal mesenchyme (HEPM) and established as a cell line. HEPM cells are plated at a low density in tissue culture dishes. After 24 hours, the test agent is added, and the cultures are maintained for an additional 72 hours without a media change. At the end of this period, the number of cells present is counted using a Coulter counter (Pratt and Willis, 1985).

Approximately 100 chemicals have been tested in this assay (Pratt and Willis, 1985; NTP, 1986; Steele et al., 1987), with and without rat liver S-9 as a metabolic activating system. Pratt and Willis (1985) reported 64% agreement with published *in vivo* results, and suggested that the HEPM test could be used as part of a battery with another test assessing a different endpoint (Pratt and Willis suggested MOT). The NTP ran the HEPM/MOT battery and reported a 72% agreement with *in vivo* results (NTP, 1986; Steele et al., 1987); however, the NTP concluded that the accuracy of the HEPM test alone was comparable to that of both tests as a battery.

Poxvirus Proliferation. The poxvirus proliferation test assesses the ability of a cell monolayer to support the growth of poxvirions. Since growth of the virus particles requires expression of the virus genome and morphogenesis of the virion, this endpoint may be developmentally relevant. BSC 40 cells infected with vaccinia WR were exposed to known teratogens and non-teratogens, and the inhibition of growth of the virus was used as an index of teratogenic potential of the test substance. Growth of the virus is assessed by counting the number of plaques (spaces on the culture plate with no cells) in each culture vessel. Fifty-one substances were screened in this system, and an 86% agreement with published *in vivo* results was reported (Keller and Smith, 1982).

Metabolic Cooperation. The metabolic cooperation assay detects intercellular communication via gap junctions. This type of cell-cell interaction is undoubtedly important in developing tissues, and interference with this may precipitate a teratogenic event. In the most widely used metabolic cooperation assay two populations of V79 cells are co-cultured, one with the ability to metabolize 6-thioguanine into a cytotoxin, the other without that ability. Under control conditions the toxic metabolite is passed between the different cell types through gap junctions, and all cells in the monolayer are killed. Under test conditions, the cells are cultured in the presence of 6-thioguanine and the test substance. If the test substance interferes with gap junctions then the passage of the toxic metabolite through them will be inhibited, and the metabolically incompetent cells will survive (Loch-Caruso and Trosko, 1985). No systematic validation of this test as a teratogen screen has been carried out, although it has been used as a screen for tumor promoters. Welsch et al. (1987) have modified this assay by using mouse limb bud cells as a model for studying the role of intercellular communication in teratogenesis.

Neuroblastoma Cell Differentiation. This screen assesses the effects of test agents on terminal differentiation of mouse neuroblastoma cells derived from malignant tumors arising originally from neural crest. Under certain culture conditions, these cells differentiate into neurons. The ability of test agents to inhibit or enhance this differentiation is evaluated. The effects of 57 test agents on differentiation of these cells have been assessed, and the reported accuracy is 86% (Mummery et al., 1983).

Primary Cultures of Embryonal Cells. Cells derived from embryos continue to undergo a number of developmental processes while in culture. This may include growth, histodifferentiation, appearance of specific gene products, etc. Thus, they may be good *in vitro* screens for substances which alter development. Although assays using primary cultures are more complex than those using established cell lines, they still typically measure a single endpoint of development; however, this may represent a composite of a number of qualitatively different developmental processes. An exception is chick embryo neural retina culture, in which individual endpoints may be evaluated as a means of gaining information about teratogenic mechanisms. These assays appear to be more powerful predictors of developmental toxicity than the established cell lines. Their disadvantages are that they require cells from living embryos, and are a little more time consuming and labor intensive than the established cell line assay systems previously discussed.

Chick Embryo Neural Crest and Limb Bud Cells. The ability of various tissues from chick embryos to differentiate in culture has been evaluated as a potential *in vitro* teratogen screen. Wilk et al. (1980) determined the sensitivity of chick embryo limb bud and neural crest cells to 14 compounds, 12 known to be teratogenic *in vivo*, and two non-teratogens. They assessed the histological differentiation of neural crest cells into neurons, and the ability of limb bud mesenchyme to express macromolecules associated with cartilage formation (proteoglycans). They reported an accuracy of 93%. Greenberg et al. (1982), from the same laboratory, described similar experiments using chick embryo neural crest cells.

Mouse Limb Bud Cells. A number of researchers have described *in vitro* developmental toxicity screens using mouse embryo limb bud cells (Hassell and Horigan, 1982; Guntakatta et al., 1984; Kistler, 1987). The cells are isolated from mouse embryo limb buds between the tenth and fourteenth days of gestation, and grown in culture in the presence of the test agent. The extent of Alcian blue staining of the culture is used as a measure of gene expression. Alcian blue stains the proteoglycans associated with cartilage matrix. Some investigators also evaluate growth, either qualitatively by staining cultures with hematoxylin and eosin (Kistler, 1987) or objectively by measuring tritiated thymidine uptake as an index of DNA synthesis (Guntakatta et al., 1984).

Guntakatta et al. (1984) reported the results of testing 22 known teratogens and 5 known non-teratogens in this system. He reported an overall accuracy of 89%, with a false negative rate of 15%. Kistler (1987) used the assay to screen a series of 25 retinoids for teratogenic activity. The potency of the retinoids in this *in vitro* system correlated very well with their *in vivo* potency for retinoids already in a biologically active form, particularly those with a free carboxylic acid group. Correlation with *in vivo* results was not good for retinoids which require metabolic activation (e.g. etretinate, motretinide). Still, this is an excellent example of the application of a test for a specific screening purpose, namely the rank ordering of a family of related chemicals for their teratogenic potency.

Drosophila Neuroblast-Myoblast Culture. The histological differentiation of Drosophila embryo neuroblasts and myoblasts in the presence of teratogens has been used as a screen (Bournias-Vardiabasis and Teplitz, 1982; Bournias-Vardiabasis et al., 1983). Neuroblasts and myoblasts are derived from embryos and cultured in the presence of the test agent. The ability to affect histological differentiation—outgrowth of neurites in the case of neuroblasts, formation of myotubes in the case of myoblasts—is evaluated microscopically. Bournias-Vardiabasis et al. (1983) tested 100 chemicals in this system, and reported an accuracy rate of 94%.

Rat Midbrain and Limb Bud Cell Culture. Flint and Orton (1984) described an *in vitro* teratogen screen which employs micromass cultures of rat embryo midbrain and limb bud cells. These are derived from gestation day 12 rat embryos, and grown in micromass culture, a procedure which concentrates the cells into a small area. The test agent is added after two hours of culture. After 5 days, differentiation is assessed by staining the limb bud cultures with Alcian blue, and the midbrain cultures with hematoxylin and eosin. Alcian blue stains cartilage matrix, and hematoxylin and eosin differentially stains differentiated and undifferentiated areas of the midbrain cultures (areas of differentiated neuronal foci stain more darkly). This scoring is made objective by using an image analyzer to quantitate staining. These authors tested 46 chemicals in this system (27 teratogens, 19 non-teratogens) in a blind protocol and reported 91% accuracy as compared to *in vivo* data.

Chick Embryo Neural Retina Cell Culture. This assay was originally developed as a model for studying tissue-specific recognition processes during development (Moscona, 1961), but has been adapted as a teratogen screen (Daston and Yonker, 1987). Neural retinas from incubation day 6 chick embryos are dissociated into single cells, then placed in a rotating culture system in the presence of the test agent for 24 hours. Under normal conditions, the cells form spherical aggregates of a specific diameter during the first several hours of culture. The cells within the aggregates form tissue layers which are comparable to those in the intact retina. Over several days in culture, cells continue to grow and divide, and differentiate. Several endpoints are quantitatively assessed, including the number and size of aggregates (a measure of cell-cell recognition and adhesion), protein content at the end of culture (an index of growth), histology of the aggregates at the end of culture (to assess histological organization and differentiation), and expression of specific proteins (to more quantitatively assess differentiation). Analysis of individual endpoints may provide mechanistic information, which may occasionally be of value in screening. Seventeen substances have been tested in this system, with an accuracy of 94% when compared to mammalian *in vivo* data (Daston et al., 1988).

Embryonic Organ Cultures. It is possible to culture embryonic organs or organ primordia. This has been done almost exclusively to study specific aspects of development in these systems, rather than for screening suspected developmental toxicants. For example, Lewis et al. (1980) and Zimmerman (1985) have cultured palatal shelves in order to investigate the biochemical and physiological factors contributing to palate closure; Kollar and Fisher (1980) have cultured tooth buds in their studies on epithelial-mesenchymal interactions in development; and fetal lung bud cultures have been used to study factors influencing the development of the pulmonary surfactant system (Doucet et al., 1987).

Limb bud cultures, first characterized by Trowell (1961) have probably been used in developmental toxicology research for the longest period. In this system, explanted rodent embryo limb buds are supported on a filter paper in a culture dish, at the interface of the medium and gas phase. Limb buds can be cultured for at least several days, during which time they grow and undergo morphological differentiation. Although this development is slower than *in vivo*, it is reproducible and consistent. This system has been used to study the effects of various teratogens on limb development (e.g. Kochhar and Aydelotte, 1974). It has been demonstrated that adult hepatic subcellular fractions (S-9 and microsomes) are compatible with limb bud culture, and are capable of activating cyclophosphamide into a moiety which is teratogenic to the limb buds (Manson and Simons, 1979).

Intact Embryos. Intact embryos of numerous species, vertebrate and invertebrate, have been advanced as being useful in screening for developmental toxicity. Intact embryos have the advantage of undergoing all of the basic processes of development, including complex interactions between heterogeneous tissue types and morphogenetic activities which may not be adequately modeled in simpler systems. Furthermore, culture of these embryos (except intact mammalian embryos) is typically uncomplicated. On the other hand, these systems have disadvantages in that they provide little information on mechanisms of teratogenesis (although this may not be a disadvantage if screening is the only intended use); many have large masses of yolk, or extra-embryonic membranes which are not comparable to those in mammals, and which may affect the quantitative delivery of test agent to the embryo; few metabolize xenobiotics in the same manner as humans, and it may be difficult or impossible to incorporate relevant metabolizing systems into most of these assays. Several intact embryos proposed as screens are phylogenetically distant from man; however, because the cellular aspects of development are highly conserved, it may be assumed that most teratogenic mechanisms acting at a cellular level are also phylogenetically comparable. On the other hand, if a substantial number of teratogens interact with receptors which are peculiar to mammals, or vertebrates, then phylogenetic distance may be important. Intact rodent embryo culture does not share many of these problems, but it does require considerable training and dexterity in the preparation of embryos for culture.

The free living embryos which have been employed most extensively in teratogen screening are the chick embryo; the embryo of the South African clawed frog, *Xenopus laevis*; the embryo of the fruit fly, *Drosophila melanogaster*; and the freshwater coelenterate, *Hydra attenuata*. Other species have been used to a lesser extent, including various fish species, brine shrimp, sea urchins and crickets.

Chick Embryos. The chick embryo has been a favorite experimental system for embryologists for centuries, and was also one of the first embryos used in experimental teratology (Dareste, 1877). This system has been adapted as a teratogen screen, and the acronym CHEST (Chick Embryotoxicity Screening Test) has been coined to define the specific protocol for the assay (Marhan and Jelinek, 1979; Jelinek, 1982).

According to this protocol, the test material is injected into the subgerminal space on incubation day 2, and into the amniotic sac on gestation days 3 and 4. Embryos are assessed for abnormal morphological development later in incubation. This protocol has been used to test 130 materials (Jelinek et al., 1985). The results correlate well with those from laboratory mammals.

A significant problem with avian embryos is that the delivery of the test agent to the embryo may be difficult to control because of the tendency for materials to distribute into the large extra-embryonic compartments of yolk and ovalbumin. This problem is minimized in the CHEST protocol, in which materials are placed in small volume fluid compartments which are directly in contact with the embryo.

Another criticism of chick embryos is that they have a limited capacity to metabolize xenobiotics (although Jelinek has demonstrated that chick embryos do possess some exogenous metabolic function), and there is no direct means to introduce a metabolizing system into the egg.

Xenopus Embryos. Various amphibian species have been used historically in experimental embryology, but developmental toxicity screening efforts directed towards assessing human risk have only been carried out in the embryos of the South African clawed frog, *Xenopus laevis*. This screening system, coined FETAX (Frog Embryo Teratogenesis Assay: Xenopus) calls for exposure of Xenopus eggs to the test agent in the water column from fertilization through the first 96 hours of development (Dumont et al., 1983). Embryos are assessed for morphological endpoints and mortality. This assay has been used by a member of researchers, and it appears to be reasonably predictive of developmental toxicity in mammals (Dumont et al., 1983; Sabourin et al., 1985; Dawson et al., 1985; Dawson and Bantle, 1987).

The drawbacks of this system include its lack of metabolizing activity, and the difficulty of testing substances which have a low solubility in water. Bantle and Dawson (1988) have added hepatic S-9 fraction from adult male rats into the aqueous medium as a xenobiotic metabolizing system, with some success.

Concerning the difficulty of testing hydrophobic materials, this is a common problem for all aquatic test systems, including *in vitro* cultures which reside in an aqueous medium. Some clever attempts have been made to overcome this problem. Sabourin (personal communication) has mixed hydrophobic materials with vegetable shortening, and added this to aquaria containing aquatic species. The hydrophobic material reaches equilibrium between the water and the shortening. The drawback to this technique is that only low concentrations of material can be tested, and it may be difficult to calculate when equilibrium is reached in the system, making it impossible to calculate actual exposure. A similar approach has been tried in rodent embryo culture, except that an emulsion is made of culture medium and corn oil containing the test material (Kitchin and Ebron, 1984). This delivery system is non-toxic to the embryo, but it is unclear what the actual exposure is from such an emulsion.

Drosophila. The fruit fly, *Drosophila melanogaster*, has been used as a developmental toxicant screen by Schuler (1982; Schuler et al., 1985), and more recently by Ranganathan et al. (1987). Fruit flies are exposed to the test material as larvae. The test agent is mixed directly with the semi-solid culture medium which serves as both food and substrate. Endpoints measured include survival to the imago (adult) stage, and the expression of external morphological abnormalities. Schuler (1982) tested seven substrates in this system, and Ranganathan et al. (1987) have tested one. The NTP is now sponsoring a validation program for this system using the 44 substances listed by the 1981 Consensus Workshop (Smith et al., 1983).

This system is attractive because it is easy to expose larvae to hydrophobic materials which form a suspension in the culture medium. Drosophila have a competent xenobiotic metabolizing system which is qualitatively similar to that in mammals, at least for polycyclic aromatic compounds (Hallstrom et al., 1984). A potential drawback to the system is the phylogenetic distance and divergence between insects and mammals.

Hydra. The freshwater coelenterate *Hydra attenuata* has been promoted by Johnson (1980) as a teratogen screen. In this assay, free-living "embryoids" are created by dissociating adult Hydra into single cells, then centrifuging these to form a cylindrical pellet, the embryoid. Over time, the embryoid organizes into an adult morph. Results of testing of over 20 materials have been published in this system (Johnson and Gabel, 1983; Johnson et al., 1984). The data derived in this system are expressed as a ratio of minimum concentration to an adult (A) to minimum developmentally toxic concentration (D). These A/D ratios are reported in lieu of absolute concentrations, and are compared with A/D ratios in mammal species, derived from reports in the literature (presumably Segment 2 studies). The relative merits of using A/D ratios to express data will be discussed later in this review. The A/D ratios reported for Hydra compare very well with mammal A/Ds. Unfortunately, these mammal studies were not specifically designed to determine minimum adult toxic dose (A); hence, few studies in the literature are suitable for calculating A/D (Rogers, 1987). Thus, it may be difficult to interpret the Hydra assay unless absolute concentrations are reported.

The drawbacks of the Hydra assay are the same as with any assay conducted in an aquatic medium: it is difficult to test hydrophobic materials, it probably has limited or no xenobiotic metabolizing capability, and it is phylogenetically distant from man. As stated above, phylogenetic distance may be insignificant given that development is highly conserved; however, the physiology of adult organisms (and hence their manifestations of toxicity) are not as highly conserved. If data from a screen are only expressed as A/D, then phylogenetic distance is potentially a concern.

Fish Embryos. A number of freshwater fish species have been used in the laboratory to test environmental chemicals for their ability to cause developmental toxicity. These include a number of North American species which have been employed by Birge and his colleagues, including fathead minnows, trout, largemouth bass and channel catfish (e.g. Birge et al., 1979). Most of these efforts have been applied to environmental toxicological screening of chemically uncharacterized industrial effluents. Thus, although embryos of these species clearly exhibit classic developmental toxic responses, there has been no rigorous validation program to determine whether they can predict human developmental toxicity. Furthermore, these species are large and often difficult to breed, and it may be difficult to maintain a large colony in most laboratories. Since the size of the aquaria must be large, a large amount of test material would be needed. The Japanese medaka fish appears to be a better candidate for reproductive toxicity screening. The medaka is a small oviparous fish which is easily obtained, cultivated and bred. Its developmental biology has been well studied, presumably because medaka embryos are remarkably transparent, making repeated non-invasive observation possible. (The zebra danio embryo has also been used as a model system in developmental biology [e.g. Eisen et al., 1986] for many of the same reasons.) The medaka has been used as a teratogen screen by Cameron et al. (1985), but these authors have only reported on the effects of lead on medaka embryos.

Other Invertebrates. Theoretically, any species could serve as an alternative screen, and many invertebrate species have been promoted for this purpose. These include planaria, sea urchins, crickets, brine shrimp, and others.

Best and Morita (1982) suggested that the ability of decapitated planaria to regenerate a head in the presence of test agents may detect teratogens. Sabourin et al. (1985) found that regeneration was affected by three of the four developmental toxicants which they tested.

Hose (1985) described an assay using sea urchin embryos which evaluates the cytotoxic, genotoxic and teratogenic effects of environmental chemicals. She reported results with only one compound, benzo(a)pyrene, a potent mutagen, but not a strong developmental toxicant. Thus, it is not possible to assess the utility of this assay for developmental toxicity screening.

The cricket has been used as a model to test the teratogenic effects of a series of polycyclic aromatic compounds (Walton, 1981; Walton et al., 1983). Cricket development appears to be very sensitive to these compounds; however, no comparisons were made to mammalian developmental toxicity.

The embryos of brine shrimp (*Artemia salina*) are susceptible to the developmental toxicity of cadmium, mercury and sodium azide (Sleet and Brendel, 1985). This species is attractive as a screen because its embryos can exist for indefinite periods in a state of anhydrobiosis, and a stock can be stored in a jar on the laboratory shelf until needed.

Rodent Embryo Culture. A procedure for the maintenance of intact post-implantation rodent embryos in culture was described by New in 1978. In this system, embryos are removed from the gravid uterus along with extra-embryonic structures. Maternal decidua and all tissue exterior to the visceral yolk sac is dissected away, and the embryo and its extra-embryonic membranes are kept in culture medium in a roller bottle for up to two days. During that period, development is roughly comparable to embryos *in situ*, although growth is considerably diminished. The quantitative response of embryos to teratogen exposures is generally comparable *in vivo* and *in vitro*; that is, abnormalities generated by a given teratogen *in utero* are also observed after addition of this material to the *in vitro* culture medium.

This assay system has been used to study various aspects of abnormal development. It is particularly useful in overcoming the complexity of the maternal system, including metabolism, distribution and excretion processes. Thus, it can be determined whether a compound requires metabolic activation, or which of a series of metabolites are teratogenic. For example, whole embryo culture has been used to demonstrate that the anti-neoplastic drug and *in vivo* teratogen cyclophosphamide has essentially no teratogenic activity, but must be metabolized to an active teratogen by monooxygenases (Fantel et al., 1979; Hales, 1981). The metabolites were then screened for teratogenic activity, and this was found to be attributable to the phosphoramide mustard metabolite (Mirkes et al., 1981), although acrolein, another metabolite, may also be embryotoxic (Mirkes et al., 1984). In a related use, Sadler and his co-workers (1985) have spent several years determining which component(s) of diabetic serum are developmentally toxic. Whole embryo culture has also been used to study the effect of teratogens which alter embryonal fluid balance (Rogers et al., 1985; Daston et al., 1987), and the effects of teratogens on visceral yolk sac function (e.g. Lloyd and Beck, 1969; Freeman and Lloyd, 1986).

At least a few laboratories have used intact rodent embryo culture as a screening system, and it is reported to correlate well with *in vivo* data (Schmid et al., 1983; Schmid, 1985; Van Malle-Fabry and Picard, 1987). Rat embryo culture has been used to detect teratogens in human serum (Chatot et al., 1980), as a possible approach to including human pharmacokinetics and metabolism in *in vitro* teratogen screening.

Rodent embryo culture may be useful in predicting the pattern of effects produced *in vivo* by a teratogen. It has been shown that *in vivo* and *in vitro* manifestations of abnormal development are similar after exposure to a number of chemicals, including hydroxyurea (Warner et al., 1983), salicylate (McGarrity et al., 1981), and trypan blue (Rogers et al., 1985).

The major disadvantage of using rodent embryo culture is that preparation of the cultures is rather labor intensive, and requires some manual dexterity, although with practice it is not a difficult technique. It is also rather expensive. Good dissecting microscopes, roller apparati, incubators and sterile hoods are among the equipment needed. The culture medium is at least 50% rat serum, and little serum can be obtained from each serum donor. However, compared to a Segment 2 study it is much less costly and time consuming and requires fewer animals. Still, it is substantially more expensive than most other *in vitro* assays.

QUANTITATIVE EXTRAPOLATIONS FROM ALTERNATIVE TESTS FOR HAZARD ASSESSMENTS

Interpretating the results from alternative test methodologies in a quantitative manner is essential since developmental toxicity is a phenomenon with a threshold, and most or all chemicals are developmentally toxic at some concentration. Since developmental toxicity is a quantitative phenomenon, it is an oversimplification to report that a substance is a developmental toxicant; instead, the concentration (or dosage) at which a substance is developmentally toxic is critical information. A number of methods for quantitatively interpretating developmental toxicity data for use in risk assessment have been proposed, and many of these may be applicable for alternative screens.

The simplest method of data interpretation is to rank compounds according to their teratogenic potency. Rankings would probably only be valid for groups of closely related compounds (congeneric series) which presumably act through a common mechanism of developmental toxicity and would have comparable pharmacokinetic properties *in vivo*. For example, Rawlings et al. (1985) used rodent whole embryo culture to generate a ranking of teratogenic potencies for the alkoxy acids (metabolites of the glycol ethers). Ranking systems could be used early in product development to select the most favorable compounds within a series for further development and future testing.

Ranking systems, although easy to construct, are not useful for determining the relationship of effective concentrations in the alternative screen to expected concentrations in *in situ* embryos, or ultimately to teratogenic doses in whole animals. The possibility exists that all members of a series may be developmentally toxic *in vivo* at the expected exposure levels, and time will have been wasted in developing these substances; or conversely, that none are developmentally toxic *in vivo* at the expected exposure levels, and useful materials will not have been developed because they were less favorably ranked. It may be possible to alleviate this problem by comparing alternative test results with those for a positive and/or negative control for which the *in vivo* developmental toxicity is known, and which have similar chemical and biological properties as the unknowns.

A second method for interpreting data is to set arbitrary upper limits of concentration for test substances. Only those substances which produce a predetermined level of toxicity at or below the arbitrary limit are considered to be developmental toxicants. The NTP used this approach in their validation study of the MOT and HEPM assays (NTP, 1986; Steele et al., 1987). As might be expected, predictive accuracy varied depending on the maximum concentration used. The highest accuracy (73%) was achieved at a 20 mM maximum concentration, and decreased at higher or lower concentrations. There were two large jumps in accuracy as the maximum concentration was increased. Percent correct was only 50% at the lowest maximum concentration used (0.05 mM), reached a plateau of approximately 65% at 0.5 mM, and increased again above 4 mM. The authors of the report propose that these changes in accuracy are due to different mechanisms of action of the test substances. At higher concentrations effects may be due to a common toxic mechanism (e.g. hypertonicity of the medium) rather than one which is pertinent to development. Although it should be possible to impose a concentration limit based on cytotoxicity, it may be difficult to detect subtle, sub-cytolethal effects which may still adversely affect parameters such as growth and differentiation. It should be noted that death of sensitive populations of cells may be a significant teratogenic event (Scott, 1977; Sulik et al., 1987); therefore, cytotoxicity may be a relevant endpoint of developmental toxicity and not a criterion of non-specific toxicity.

For intact embryos, it has been proposed that ratios of adult to developmental toxicity may be used as a means of assessing levels of hazard. Fabro et al. (1982) and Johnson (1981) have proposed similar schemes for calculating these ratios. Fabro et al. (1982) have advocated the use of a relative teratogenic index (RTI), calculated by dividing the adult LD-01 by the teratogenic dose (tD)-05. Johnson (1981) has proposed the A/D ratio, which is the adult toxic LOEL divided by the LOEL for developmental toxicity. He has modified this recently to be calculated as adult NOEL/developmental NOEL (Johnson, 1987). Both are based on the concept that most teratogenic hazards are specifically toxic to the embryo and are far more potent developmental toxicants than adult toxicants. These substances would have a high RTI or A/D, and would be significant reproductive hazards. In practice, this concept may not be true, since many human teratogens (e.g. chemotherapeutic agents, anti-convulsants, ethanol) are only teratogenic at or near levels which cause maternal toxicity.

It is significant that both indices make use of the lowest toxic dose levels rather than LD-50 or tD-50. Because the dose-response curves for each toxic phenomenon may differ significantly in slope, ratios of LD-50 to tD-50 may be substantially different than ratios of lower incidence levels. Unfortunately, the confidence limits at the low end of dose-response curves tend to be large; therefore, there is much greater uncertainty in the actual values for concentrations which produce few effects.

Although RTI and A/D are fundamentally similar, they differ in that RTI is a statistical value calculated from a dose-response curve, whereas A/D is a ratio of LOELs, with no consideration given to the slope of the dose-response curve. Johnson, the developer of the A/D concept, has not published a statistical treatment of A/D data. Instead, he has established a critical A/D ratio of 3, above which there is substantial concern of reproductive hazard, and below which there is less concern (Johnson et al., 1987).

Thus far, the RTI has only been used on data generated in laboratory mammals (Fabro et al., 1982). The A/D ratio has been used to compare developmental toxicity generated in Hydra with mammalian data, and it has been proposed from these comparisons that A/D is consistent across species (Johnson and Gabel, 1983). Since A/D and RTI are similar, it is possible that either could be used to determine developmental hazard from screens which use alternative species. However, there is some doubt that A/D is constant across species in all cases (Rogers, 1987), and Johnson's mammalian A/D's may not be completely accurate (Brown, 1986). At the very least, the constancy of A/D should be verified in several alternative species before it is accepted as a general principle. The A/D ratio may also be more useful if a standardized criterion for minimum adult toxicity (e.g. LD-05) were adopted for all species.

A ratio of embryolethality to teratogenicity, called the teratogenic index, has been used as a means of ranking teratogenic hazard in the Xenopus embryo assay (Dumont et al., 1983). This ratio may be useful in distinguishing between teratogens and embryotoxins, but since both endpoints are manifestations of developmental toxicity, the ratios will not be useful in extrapolating alternative data for hazard assessment.

Finally, it may be possible to design alternative screens such that they utilize *in vivo* pharmacokinetic data to set concentration levels in the alternative system. The conversion of mg/kg dose levels in pregnant mammals to μg/ml concentrations in *in vitro* screens is an example of the crudest use of pharmacokinetic principles in selecting concentrations for these screens. Unfortunately, mg/kg dosage is often very different from μg/ml concentration at the embryo, or in the maternal serum which comes into contact with the extra-embryonic tissues. A slightly more sophisticated method of concentration selection would be to estimate the volume of distribution of the test compound based on its physical and chemical properties (e.g. water solubility, molecular weight, charge) although for highly lipophilic materials even this is impractical. The optimum method, is to empirically determine the peak serum concentration or peak embryo concentration in a pregnant lab animal produced by a toxic dose (e.g. an LD-05) of the test chemical. This would serve as an upper limit of concentration in an *in vitro* assay. Toxicity in the alternative assay at higher concentrations would not be relevant because those concentrations would not be achieved *in situ*. A pharmacokinetic approach would probably not be routine, but might be desirable if the *in vitro* data were to be the sole basis for risk assessment. Even this approach is not foolproof, however. There may be considerable differences in the pharmacokinetic properties of an *in vitro* system as compared to the embryo *in utero*. *In vivo* there is a continual removal of the test chemical from the maternal circulation, either by metabolism, elimination or distribution to tissues. *In vitro* no such removal occurs; thus, the *in vitro* system is exposed to the maximum concentration of test chemical or its metabolites for the entire period of exposure. If duration of exposure is significant to the material's toxicity, it may be possible to reach a threshold *in vitro* which would not have been reached *in vivo*. There are examples of chemicals for which duration of exposure (area under the exposure curve) is significant, and conversely of chemicals in which peak exposure level is far more important in determining toxicity (Nau, 1987).

Binding of teratogens to serum proteins may also be important in the degree to which they interact with the embryo. *In vitro* culture media is lower in protein concentration than whole serum (media is typically 10-50% serum). Decreased serum protein concentration may result in a higher percentage of chemical free to interact with the target tissue. Schmid et al. (1987) have shown that the dose response relationship for the teratogenicity of aspirin in rat embryo culture depends both on the amount of serum in the medium and the vehicle in which the aspirin is dissolved.

Considering matters of elimination or protein binding, *in vitro* systems would be expected to be more sensitive to teratogens than the embryo *in utero*; thus, errors would be on the side of caution.

POTENTIAL APPLICATION OF *IN VITRO* TERATOGEN SCREENS IN SAFETY ASSESSMENT

The eventual goal of *in vitro* methods development is to employ these tests in the safety assessment of new pharmaceutical, commercial, industrial, and agricultural chemicals. Of course, the intended use of the new chemical will influence the testing scheme to which it is subjected, and the relative placement and significance of *in vitro* assays in that scheme. For example, it is not possible now (and perhaps never) to substitute *in vitro* tests for *in vivo* assessments of developmental toxicity for materials intended to be administered to humans or which will have widespread environmental use. On the other hand, it may be possible to use *in vitro* tests to screen large series of related candidate drugs to select only the ones with low teratogenic potential for further *in vivo* testing. In cases where exposure to materials is limited, and exposure concentrations are low, *in vitro* tests may play an increasingly important role in assessment. For many industrial chemicals there is no routine testing for developmental toxicity. Employing rapid and reliable *in vitro* assays to screen such materials would be of great benefit.

There are specific instances where *in vitro* assays may be of immediate use in predicting teratogenic potential of new compounds. We have previously cited the work of Kistler (1987) in which he demonstrated that there is an excellent correlation between the sensitivity of *in vivo* mouse limb bud cells and *in situ* embryos to the teratogenicity of a series of retinoids. This *in vitro* system is sensitive to the teratogenic mechanism of the retinoids and can correctly rank them as to their teratogenic potential. Although it would certainly be necessary to test materials such as retinoids which are intended for pharmaceutical application *in vivo*, this approach could at least limit the number of compounds needing to be tested *in vivo* from tens or hundreds to just a few.

In vitro screens may be of greater importance in screening materials for which standard developmental toxicity screening is not typically done, including industrial chemicals for which exposure is limited. In such instances, *in vitro* screening may be the only approach which is economically feasible. Of course, it will be necessary to demonstrate that the *in vitro* tests used are reliable before they are applied for general use.

As more *in vitro* assays are demonstrated to be effective at predicting teratogenesis, it may become feasible to construct a battery or tiered system for using *in vitro* screens. Batteries may be useful if it is determined that a series of simple *in vitro* assays are better at predicting teratogenic potential than a single assay. This approach is attractive when one considers that a battery can be constructed in which each segment assesses a different developmental endpoint and therefore detects a different teratogenic mechanism. In practice, it will need to be demonstrated by standardized validation programs that combinations of tests are in fact more accurate than single tests. Thus far, the only attempt to do this demonstrated that the MOT and HEPM tests together were not more predictive than the HEPM test alone (NTP, 1986), even though it was believed that the battery would be more predictive (Pratt and Willis, 1985). Although this result is interesting, it is insufficiently comprehensive to permit us to conclude that a battery approach will not be effective.

In lieu of a battery, a tiered approach may be an efficient means of screening for teratogenic potential. The first tier of testing could be one of the assays using primary cultures of embryonal cells or intact sub-mammalian embryos, which appear to be reasonably predictive. If this test is negative at testing concentrations which are higher than expected from calculated (e.g., by volume of distribution) or empirically measured peak concentrations *in vivo* then the material can be considered to pose no developmental risk. The second tier would be rodent embryo culture. Again, if the material produces no adverse effects at or above biological relevant concentrations, then it need not be tested further. If it does produce adverse effects, then standard *in vivo* testing would have to be carried out in order to appropriately quantitate the risk.

CONCLUSIONS

In vitro teratogen screens are intended to be simple models of *in vivo* development, which are easy to carry out and interpret. Many of these models were developed as tools for studying specific teratogenic mechanisms, and have been useful for this purpose. There have been numerous studies using whole embryo, organ, and primary embryonal cell cultures which have added to our knowledge of basic events in normal and abnormal development. Many *in vitro* systems have been adapted as teratogen screens, along with several assays using established cell lines which were expressly developed for screening. Validation programs have been carried out for a number of these screens. It is clear from these efforts that the most effective validation programs are standardized, take place in laboratories independent of the one developing the assay, and take into account the quantitative relationship between administered concentration and developmental toxicity.

There are currently a few practical uses for *in vitro* teratogenicity assays. They will continue to be extremely useful in studying mechanisms of teratogenesis. There are also instances in which some of these assays may be of immediate use in screening. In particular, *in vitro* screens may be used to rank chemically related families of compounds for their relative teratogenic potencies. It is only necessary that the test used be shown to be sensitive to the mechanism of toxicity through which this series of chemicals exerts its developmental toxicity. Examples of successful uses of *in vitro* screens for this purpose include a rank ordering of retinoids (Kistler, 1987) and glycol ether metabolites (Rawlings et al., 1985).

Use of these assays for more general screening purposes may not be possible yet, unless an unknown (and perhaps large) error rate is acceptable, and further testing in more traditional assays is planned. Of course, acceptable error rates will vary depending on the intended use of the test, and the gravity assigned to a positive response in such a test will be a function of its record of accuracy. It is possible that even tests with a relatively high error rate will still be of some value in the early stages of safety assessments. A number of the short term genetic toxicity screens have high error rates, but still provide useful information and increase the level of confidence that a material is correctly classified by another more reliable method.

Any generic use of *in vitro* teratogen screens will require a certain level of knowledge about the predictiveness, peculiarities and specific shortcomings of each *in vitro* test. We hope that effort will continue in validating and refining these assays so that they will eventually be of use in safety assessments. It will also be important to continue to establish methods for quantitatively interpreting data from *in vitro* screens. This may include adapting expressions of relative potency, such as the A/D ratio or RTI, to *in vitro* systems, or may involve more extensive research on comparative pharmacokinetics of the *in vivo* mammal embryo and *in vitro* systems. The pharmacokinetic approach will be difficult, but has the potential to be of greatest use in interpretating data generated *in vitro* and ultimately applying it to human risk assessment.

REFERENCES

BANTLE, J.A. and DAWSON, D.A. (1988). Uninduced rat liver microsomes as a metabolic activating system for the frog embryo teratogenesis assay—Xenopus (FETAX), in Aquatic Toxicology and Hazard Assessment, vol. 10 (W.J. Adams, G.A. Chapman and W.G. Lindis, eds.), American Society for Testing and Materials STP 971, Philadelphia, in press.

BEST, J.B. and MORITA, M. (1982). Planarians as a model system for *in vitro* teratogenesis studies. Teratogen. Carcinogen. Mutagen. **2**:277–291.

BIRGE, W.J., BLACK, J.A., WESTERMAN, A.G. and RAMEY, B.A. (1983). Fish and amphibian embryos—a model system for evaluating teratogenicity. Fund. Appl. Toxicol. **3**:237–242.

BOURNIAS-VARDIABASIS, N., TEPLITZ, R.L., CHERNOFF, G.F. and SEECOF, R.L. (1983). Detection of teratogens in the Drosophila embryonic cell culture test: Assay of 100 chemicals. Teratology **28**:109–122.

BOURNIAS-VARDIABASIS, N. and TEPLITZ, R.L. (1982). Use of Drosophila embryo cell cultures as an *in vitro* teratogen assay. Teratogen. Carcinogen. Mutagen. 2.

BRAUN, A.G., BUCKNER, C.A., EMERSON, D.J. and NICHISON, B.B. (1982). Quantitative correspondence between the *in vitro* activity of teratogenic agents. Proc. Natl. Acad. Sci. USA **79**:2056–2060.

BRAUN, A.G., EMERSON, D.J. and NICHISON, B.B. (1979). Teratogenic drugs inhibit tumor cell attachment to lectin-coated surfaces. Nature **282**:507–509.

BRAUN, A.G. and HOROWICZ, P.B. (1983). Lectin-mediated attachment assay for teratogens: Results with 32 pesticides. J. Toxicol. Environ. Health **11**:275–286.

BROWN, L.P., FLINT, O.P., ORTON, T.C. and GIBSON, G.G. (1986). Chemical teratogenesis: Testing methods and the role of metabolism. Drug Metab. Rev. **17**:221–260.

BROWN, N.A. (1986). Alternative tests for teratogenicity of petroleum products. Critical review prepared for the American Petroleum Institute.

BROWN, N.A. and KRAM, D. (1982). Intact human and rodent hepatic cells used for bioactivation in an embryo culture system. Teratology **25**:30A.

CAMERON, I.L., LAWRENCE, W.C. and LUM, J.B. (1985). Medaka eggs as a model system for screening potential teratogens, in Prevention of Physical and Mental Congenital Defects, Part C: Basic and Medical Science, Education, and Future Strategies, Alan R. Liss, New York, pp. 239–243.

CHATOT, C.L., KLEIN, N.W., PIATEK, J. and PIERRO, L.J. (1980). Successful culture of rat embryos on human serum: Use in the detection of teratogens. Science **207**:1471–1473.

DARESTE, C. (1877). Recherches sur la production artificielle des monstruosites, ou Essais de teratogenie experimentale. C. Reinwald, Paris.

DASTON, G.P., EBRON, M.T., CARVER, B. and STEFANANDIS, J.G. (1987). *In vitro* teratogenicity of ethylenethiourea in the rat. Teratology **35**:239–245.

DASTON, G.P. and YONKER, J.E. (1987). Chick embryo retina cell culture as an *in vitro* teratogen screen. The Toxicologist **7**:141.

DASTON, G.P., YONKER, J.E., BAINES, D. and POYNTER, J.I. (1988). Chick embryo retina cell culture: Teratogen screen and mechanistic probe. The Toxicologist **8**:114.

DASTON, G.P., YONKER, J.E. and POWERS, J.F. (1987). Studies of the teratogenicity of ETU to rat and mouse embryos *in vitro*. Teratology **35**:72A–73A.

DAWSON, D.A. and BANTLE, J.A. (1987). Coadministration of methylxanthines and inhibitor compounds potentiates teratogenicity in Xenopus embryos. Teratology **35**:221–227.

DAWSON, D.A., McCORMICK, C.A. and BANTLE, J.A. (1985). Detection of teratogenic substances in acidic mine water samples using the frog embryo teratogenesis assay—Xenopus (FETAX). J. Appl. Toxicol. **5**:234–244.

DOUCET, E., BURBON, J., RIEUTORT, M., MARIN, L. and TORDET, C. (1987). Optimization of fetal lung organ culture for surfactant biosynthesis. *In vitro* Cell. Devel. Biol. **23**:189–198.

DUMONT, J.N., SCHULTZ, T.W., BUCHANAN, M. and KAO, G. (1983). Frog embryo teratogenesis assay: Xenopus (FETAX)—A short-term assay applicable to complex environmental mixtures. In: Symposium on the Application of Short-Term Bioassays in the Analysis of Complex Environmental Mixtures, M.D., Waters, S.S. Sandhu, J. Lewtas, L. Claxton, and S. Nesnow, eds. Plenum Press, New York, pp. 393–405.

EISEN, J.S., MYERS, P.Z. and WESTERFIELD, M. (1986). Pathway selection by growth cones of identified motoneurons in live zebrafish embryos. Nature **320**:269–271.

FABRO, S., SHULL, G. and BROWN, N.A. (1982). The relative teratogenic index and teratogenic potency: Proposed components of developmental toxicity risk assessment. Teratogen. Carcinogen. Mutagen. **2**:61–76.

FANTEL, A.G., GREENAWAY, J.C., JUCHAU, M.R. and SHEPHARD, T.H. (1979). Teratogenic bioactivation of cyclophosphamide *in vitro*. Life Sci. **25**:67–72.

FLINT, O.P. and ORTON, T.C. (1984). An *in vitro* assay for teratogens with cultures of rat embryo midbrain and limb bud cells. Toxicol. Appl. Pharmacol. **76**:383–395.

FREEMAN, S.J. and LLOYD, J.B. (1986). Evidence that suramin and aurothiomalate are teratogenic in rat by disturbing yolk sac-mediated embryonic protein nutrition. Chem.-Biol. Interactions **58**:149–160.

GREENBERG, J.H. (1982). Detection of teratogens by differentiating embryonic neural crest cells in culture: Evaluation as a screening system. Teratogen. Carcinogen. Mutagen. **2**:319–323.

GUNTAKATTA, M., MATTHEWS, E.J. and RUNDELL, J.O. (1984). Development of a mouse embryo limb bud cell culture system for the estimation of chemical teratogenic potential. Teratogen. Carcinogen. Mutagen. **4**:349–364.

HALES, B.F. (1981). Modification of the mutagenicity and teratogenicity of cyclophosphamide in rats with inducers of the cytochromes P-450. Teratology **24**:1–11.

HALLSTROM, I., BLANCK, A. and ATUMA, S. (1984). Genetic variation in cytochrome P-450 and xenobiotic metabolism in Drosophila melanogaster. Biochem. Pharmacol. **33**:13–20.

HASSELL, J.R. and HORIGAN, E.A. (1982). Chondrogenesis: A model developmental system for measuring teratogenic potential of compouneds. Teratogen. Carcinogen. Mutagen. **2**:325–331.

HOSE, J.E. (1985). Potential uses of sea urchin embryos for identifying toxic chemicals: Description of a bioassay incorporating cytologic, cytogenetic and embryologic endpoints. J. Appl. Toxicol. **5**:245–254.

JELINEK, R. (1982). Use of chick embryo in screening for embryotoxicity. Teratogen. Carcinogen. Mutagen. **2**:255–261.

JELINEK, R., PETERKA, M. and RYCHTER, Z. (1985). Chick embryotoxicity screening test—130 substances tested. Indian J. Exp. Biol. **23**:588–595.

JOHNSON, E.M. (1980). A subvertebrate system for rapid determination of potential teratogenic hazards. J. Environ. Pathol. Toxicol. **4**:153–156.

JOHNSON, E.M. (1981). Screening for teratogenic hazards: Nature of the problems. Ann. Rev. Pharmacol. Toxicol. **21**:417–429.

JOHNSON, E.M. (1987). A tier system for developmental toxicity evaluations based on considerations of exposure and effect relationships. Teratology **35**:405–427.

JOHNSON, E.M., CHRISTIAN, M.S. (1984). When is a teratology study not an evaluation of teratogenicity? J. Amer. Coll. Toxicol. **3**:431–434.

JOHNSON, E.M., CHRISTIAN, M.S., DANSKY, L. and GABEL, B.E.G. (1987). Use of the adult developmental relationship in prescreening for developmental hazards. Teratogen. Carcinogen. Mutagen. **7**:273–285.

JOHNSON, E.M. and GABEL, B.E.G. (1983). An artificial "embryo" for detection of abnormal development. Fundam. Appl. Toxicol. **3**:243–249.

JOHNSON, E.M., GABEL, B.E.G. and LARSON, J. (1984). Developmental toxicity and structure/activity correlates of glycols and glycol ethers. Environ. Health Perspect. **57**:135–139.

KELLER, S.J. and SMITH, M.K. (1982). Animal virus screens for potential teratogens. I. Poxvirus morphogenesis. Teratogen. Carcinogen. Mutagen. **2**:361–374.

KIMMEL, G.L., SMITH, K., KOCHHAR, D.M. and PRATT, R.M. (1982). Overview of *in vitro* teratogenicity testing: Aspects of validation and application to screening. Teratogen. Carcinogen. Mutagen. **2**:221–229.

KISTLER, A. (1987). Limb bud cell cultures for estimating the teratogenic potential of compounds. Arch. Toxicol. **60**:403–414.

KITCHIN, K.T. and EBRON, M.T. (1984). Further development of rodent whole embryo culture: Solvent toxicity and water insoluble compound delivery system. Toxicology **30**:45–57.

KITCHIN, K.T., SCHMID, B.P. and SANYAL, M.K. (1981). Teratogenicity of cyclophosphamide in a coupled microsomal activating/embryo culture system. Biochem. Pharmacol. **30**:59–64.

KOCHHAR, D.M. and AYDELOTTE, M.B. (1974). Susceptible stages and abnormal morphogenesis in the developing mouse limb, analyzed in organ culture after transplacental exposure to vitamin A (retinoic acid). J. Embryol. Exper. Morphol. **31**:721–734.

KOLLAR, E.J. and FISHER, C. (1980). Tooth induction in chick epithelium: Expression of quiescent genes for enamel synthesis. Science **207**:993–995.

LEWIS, C.A., THIBAULT, L., PRATT, R.M. and BRINKLEY, L.L. (1980). An improved culture system for secondary palatal evaluation. *In Vitro* **16**:453–460.

LLOYD, J.B. and BECK, F. (1969). Teratogenesis, in Lysosomes in Biology and Pathology, vol. 1 (J.T. Dingle and H.B. Fell, eds.), North Holland, Amsterdam, pp. 433–449.

LOCH-CARUSO, R. and TROSKO, J.E. (1985). Inhibited intercellular communication as a mechanistic link between teratogenesis and carcinogenesis. CRC Crit. Rev. Toxicol. **16**:157–183.

MANSON, J.M. and SIMONS, R. (1979). *In vitro* metabolism of cyclophosphamide in limb bud culture. Teratology **19**:149–158.

MARHAN, O. and JELINEK, R. (1979). Efficiency of embryotoxicity testing procedures. II. Comparison between the official, MEST and CHEST methods. Toxicol. Lett. **4**:389–392.

McGARRITY, C., SAMANI, N., BECK, F. and GULAMHUSEIM, A. (1981). The effect of sodium salcylate on the rat embryo in culture: An *in vitro* model for the morphological assessment of teratogenicity. J. Anat. **133**:257–269.

MIRKES, P.E., FANTEL, A.G., GREENAWAY, J.C. and SHEPHARD, T.H. (1981). Teratogenicity of cyclophosphamide metabolites: Phosphoramide mustard, acrolein and 4-ketocyclophosphamide in rat embryos cultured *in vitro*. Toxicol. Appl. Pharmacol. **58**:322–330.

MIRKES, P.E., GREENAWAY, J.C., ROGERS, J.G. and BRUNDRETT, R.B. (1984). Role of acrolein in cyclophosphamide teratogenicity in rat embryos *in vitro*. Toxicol. Appl. Pharmacol. **72**:281–291.

MOSCONA, A. (1961). Rotation-mediated histogenetic aggregation of dissociated cells. Exper. Cell Res. **22**:455–475.

NAU, H. (1987). Species differences in pharmacokinetics, drug metabolism, and teratogenesis, in Pharmacokinetics in Teratogenesis, vol. 1 (H. Nau and W.J. Scott, Jr., eds.), CRC Press, Boca Raton, FL, pp. 81–106.

NEW, D.A.T. (1978). Whole embryo culture and the study of mammalian embryos during organogenesis. Biol. Review **53**:81–122.

NTP (1986). Evaluation of two *in vitro* teratology test systems. Final report. National Toxicology Program, National Institute of Environmental Health Sciences, NTP-86-372.

OGLESBY, L.A., EBRON, M.T., BEYER, P.E., CARVER, B.D. and KAVLOCK, R.J. (1986). Co-culture of rat embryos and hepatocytes: *In vitro* detection of a proteratogen. Teratogen. Carcinogen. Mutagen. **6**:129–138.

PRATT, R.M. and WILLIS, W.D. (1985). *In vitro* screening assay for teratogens using growth inhibition of human embryonic cells. Proc. Natl. Acad. Sci. USA **82**:5791–5794.

RANGANATHAN, S., DAVIS, D.G. and HOOD, R.D. (1987). Developmental toxicity of ethanol in *Drosophila melanogaster*. Teratology **36**:45–49.

RAWLINGS, S.J., SHUKER, D.E.G., WEBB, M. and BROWN, N.A. (1985). The teratogenic potential of alkoxy acids in post-implantation rat embryo culture: Structure-activity relationships. Toxicol. Letters **28**:49–58.

ROGERS, J.M. (1987). Comparison of maternal and fetal toxic dose responses in mammals. Teratogen. Carcinogen. Mutagen. **7**:297–306.

ROGERS, J.M., DASTON, G.P., EBRON, M.T., CARVER, B., STEFANADIS, J.G. and GRABOWSKI, C.T. (1985). Studies on the mechanism of trypan blue teratogenicity *in vivo* and *in vitro*. Teratology **31**:389–399.

SABOURIN, T.D., FAULK, R.T. and GOSS, L.B. (1985). The efficacy of three non-mammalian test systems in the identification of chemical teratogens. J. Appl. Toxicol. **5**:227–233.

SADLER, T.W., HORTON, W.E. and HUNTER, E.S. (1985). Mammalian embryos in culture: A new approach to investigating normal and abnormal developmental mechanisms, in Developmental Mechanisms: Normal and Abnormal, Alan R. Liss, New York, pp. 227–240.

SCHMID, B.P. (1985). Teratogenicity testing of new drugs with the postimplantation embryo culture system, in *In Vitro* Embrytoxicity and Teratogenicity Tests (F. Homburger and A.M. Goldberg, eds.), S. Karger, Basel, pp. 46–57.

SCHMID, B.P., CIRCUREL, L. and MARAZZI, A. (1987). Correlation between drug concentrations and teratogenicity *in vivo* and *in vitro*, in Pharmacokinetics in Teratogenesis, vol. 2 (H. Nau and W.J. Scott, Jr., eds.). CRC Press, Boca Raton, FL, pp. 209–217.

SCHMID, B.P., TRIPPMACHER, A. and BIANCHI, A. (1983). Validation of the whole-embryo culture method for *in vitro* teratogenicity testing, in Developments in the Science and Practice of Toxicology (A.W. Hayes, R.C. Schnell and T.S. Miya, eds.), Elsevier, Amsterdam, pp. 563–566.

SCHULER, R.L., HARDIN, B.D. and NIEMEIER, R.W. (1982). Drosophila as a tool for the rapid assessment of chemicals for teratogenicity. Teratogen. Carcinogen. Mutagen. **2**:293–301.

SCHULER, R.L., RADIKE, M.A., HARDIN, B.D. and NIEMEIER, R.W. (1985). Pattern of response of intact Drosophila to known teratogens. J. Amer. Coll. Toxicol. **4**:291–303.

SCOTT, W.J. (1977). Cell death and reduced proliferative rate, in Handbook of Teratology, vol. 2 (J.G. Wilson and F.C. Fraser, eds.), Plenum, New York, pp. 81–98.

SHEPARD, T.H., FANTEL, A.G., MIRKES, P.E., GREENAWAY, J.C., FAUSTMAN-WATTS, E., CAMPBELL, M. and JUCHAU, M.R. (1983). Teratology testing. I. Development and status of short-term prescreens. II. Biotransformation of teratogens as studied in whole embryo culture. Devel. Pharmacol. **1**:147–164.

SHUM, S., JENSEN, N.M. and NEBERT, D.W. (1979). The Ah locus: In utero toxicity and teratogenesis associated with genetic differences in benzo(a)pyrene metabolism. Teratology **20**:365–376.

SLEET, R.B. and BRENDEL, K. (1985). Homogeneous populations of Artemia nauplii and their potential use for *in vitro* testing in developmental toxicology. Teratogen. Carcinogen. Mutagen. **5**:41–54.

SMITH, M.K., KIMMEL, G.L., KOCHHAR, D.M., SHEPARD, T.H., SPIELBERG, S.P. and WILSON, J.G. (1983). A selection of candidate compounds for *in vitro* teratogenesis test validation. Teratogen. Carcinogen. Mutagen. **3**:461–480.

STEELE, V.E., MORRISSEY, R.E., LAMB, J.C., WILKINSON, B.P., ROCHA, D.G., MURPHY, D.D. and ELMORE, E.L. (1987). Evaluation of two *in vitro* assays to screen for potential teratogens. 1987 EMS Abstracts: **103**.

SULIK, K.K., JOHNSTON, M.C. and DEHART, D.B. (1987). Potentiation of programmed cell death by 13-cis retinoic acid: A common mechanism for early craniofacial and limb malformations? Teratology **35**:32A.

TROWELL, O.A. (1961). Problems in the maintenance of mature organs *in vitro*, in La Culture Organotypique, Editions du Centre Nationale de la Recherche Scientifique, Paris, 1961, pp. 237–249.

WALTON, B.T. (1981). Chemical impurity produces extra compound eyes and heads in crickets. Science **212**:51–53.

WALTON, B.T., HO, C.-H., MA, C.Y., O'NEILL, E.G. and KAO, G.L. (1983). Benzoquino-linediones: Activity as insect teratogens. Science **222**:422–423.

WARNER, C.W., SADLER, T.W., SHOCKEY, J. and SMITH, M.K. (1983). A comparison of the *in vivo* and *in vitro* response of mammalian embryos to a teratogenic insult. Toxicology **28**:271–282.

WELSCH, F., STEDMAN, D.B. and CARSON, J.L. (1987). Teratogen interference with cell interactions: Cell-to-cell channel disruption as a potential mechanism of abnormal development. In: Approaches to Elucidate Mechanisms in Teratogenesis, F. Welsch, ed. Hemisphere Pub. Co., Washington, D.C., in press.

WILK, A.L., GREENBERG, J.H., HORIGAN, E.A., PRATT, R.M. and MARTIN, G.R. (1980). Detection of teratogenic compounds using differentiating embryonic cells in culture. *In Vitro* **16**:269–276.

WILSON, J.G. (1973). Environment and Birth Defects, Academic, New York.

ZIMMERMAN, E.F. (1985). Role of neurotransmitters in palate development and teratogenic implications, in Developmental Mechanisms: Normal and Abnormal. Alan R. Liss, New York, pp. 283–294.

IN VITRO SCREENS FROM CNS, LIVER AND KIDNEY FOR SYSTEMIC TOXICITY

CHARLES A. TYSON* AND NEILL H. STACEY†

***SRI International**
Menlo Park, California

†National Institute of Occupational Health and Safety
The University of Sydney
Sydney, Australia

The development and evaluation of in vitro *systems from target organs for preliminary assessments of the potential for systemic toxic effects has been receiving increased attention. This review presents a synopsis of progress made in developing toxicity screens for three common target organs and identifies further work needed for more complete validation.*

INTRODUCTION

Most foreign chemicals taken into the body in sufficient amount can produce systemic effects or toxicity. These chemicals exert their effects ordinarily on a limited number of internal organs, so-called target organs. Common internal target organs are the central nervous system, blood and the hematopoietic system, liver, kidney, and lung (Klaassen, 1986). Functional impairment may ensue from a brief, prolonged or

---

1. Address correspondence to: Dr. Charles A. Tyson, SRI International, Menlo Park, CA 94025.
2. Key words: central nervous system, hepatocyte, kidney tubule.

repeated exposure to the chemical. Severe compromise of the cell's capability for conducting normal functions is considered a cytotoxic response. The ultimate result may be any number of pathologic conditions, including cell death or that of the organism, depending on the nature of the exposure and the injury.

An important application for *in vitro* systems is the preliminary screening of xenobiotics for potential systemic effects. For the greatest confidence in the results there is no fully satisfactory alternative to using tissues from common target organs or the suspected targets, as no single cell type can be substituted. The HeLa cell system, for example, gives a good correspondence between *in vitro* IC_{50} and *in vivo* lethal dosages in mice or humans for the majority of chemicals evaluated but significantly underestimates the toxic potential of potent neurospecific drugs (Ekwall, 1980a, b, c). Ekwall and Acosta (1982) found that four of 14 hepatotoxic chemicals *in vivo* were more toxic to hepatocytes in suspension or monolayer culture than either HeLa or Chang liver cells. The chemicals that produced lesser responses in the cell lines are thought to require metabolic activation for toxicity *in vivo*. Gray and Beamand (1984) and Gray et al. (1985) developed a primary mixed culture of rat testicular cells and showed that the same target cells as *in vivo* for phthalate esters (Sertoli) and for alkoxyacetic acid metabolites of glycol ethers (dividing spermatocytes, as well as the pachytene) were selectively affected.

The present review is an abbreviated synopsis of progress in the development of *in vitro* systems from three common target organs for screening purposes. These systems have the theoretical and in some cases actual benefit of reducing animal usage and costs for testing. Brain, liver, and kidney are chosen for review here, because these targets offer a variety of difficulties in replicating effects on them in *in vitro* preparations. The stress here is on studies where cellular response of several chemicals has been evaluated and compared with relative potency *in vivo*. Other reviews related to this topic appear in Acosta et al. (1985), Shakar and Goldberg (1987), Rauckman and Padilla (1987), Fisher and Placke (1987), Placke and Fisher (1987), Gardner et al. (1988), and McQueen (in press).

CENTRAL NERVOUS SYSTEM (CNS)

Test systems development for this target system is for the most part in its relative infancy. The complexity of neurological tissues and processes and the existence of the blood-brain barrier offer unique problems for this application. Since nerve function and tissues are targets for many chemicals at low doses, screens that identify potential neurotoxicants would be very valuable.

Approaches that are being developed and evaluated include noncellular (myelin- or transmitter-related enzyme assays like cholinesterase, receptor binding or mediated events), cellular (disperse primary cultures, reaggregated cultures, cell lines) or tissue (organotypic cultures, brain slices). Suspensions of enriched microvessels and cerebral endothelial cells grown on collagen or formed into sheets separating compartments in a Ussing chamber offer *in vitro* models of promise for studies of blood-brain barrier transport properties (Bradbury, 1985). One can envision ultimately the construct of coculture systems of neuronal cells or structural components from different CNS regions surrounded by endothelial cell monolayers that would reproduce site-specific alterations modulated by the presence of a simulated blood-brain barrier.

When action of a chemical class of neurotoxicants is known and specific for a particular neuronal component, relatively simple test systems can be developed that provide reliable results even for the human situation. A now-classic example is the discrimination of acute from delayed neurotoxic effects of organophosphorus compounds possible by assaying neurotoxic esterase and acetylcholinesterase in hen brain homogenates exposed to the compounds (Johnson, 1977; Lotti and Johnson, 1978). Since receptors are involved in many pharmacologic and pathologic phenomena, assays of the effects of neurotoxic agents on receptor binding too may be valid and sensitive.

On this supposition, Bondy (1982) proposed a receptor-ligand screening system in which several receptors involved in neural circuits from different brain regions are assayed. Pharmacologic agents are substituted for the presumptive endogenous receptor ligands in the assays. The assays require little tissue and time to complete, and thus could be economical, a concern for tissue-culture approaches (Dewar, 1981). Disturbances in binding phenomena are reported for several neurotoxicants, including both organic molecules and metal ions. Much learning is required, as Bondy notes, to be able to discriminate potentially toxicologic from pharmacologic, or relatively innocuous, responses in assays of this kind, but their simplicity merits continued interest. For example, measurements of muscarinic cholinergic receptors in the caudate nucleus in conjunction with acetylcholinesterase assays discriminated between effects of organophosphates and carbamates at low and high concentrations, which is of possible relation to the chronic and acute effects of these chemicals *in vivo* (Volpe et al., 1985).

More general interest has centered on developing cellular or tissue neurotoxicity screens, despite acknowledged difficulties. Some intriguing possibilities exist (Shakar and Goldberg, 1987), but many are still in the early stage of development and characterization. Among older approaches available, brain slices and neuroblastoma and cell line cultures have either still to be tested systematically (Fountain and Teyler, 1987), require caution in interpreting results (Smith et al., 1987), or yield results inconsistent with modulation of cholinergic receptor expression *in vivo*, a prerequisite for target selectivity (Clementi et al., 1987).

A fair amount of data has accumulated, however, to consider organotypic neural cultures as models and testing systems for both acute and subchronic chemical-induced neurotoxicity (Whetsell and Schwarz, 1984; Spencer et al., 1986). The systems are developed from explants of motor and/or sensory neural components maturing in cultures. Explants from most regions of the brain have been successfully cultured. A number of cocultures, for example, fetal mouse spinal cord and dorsal root ganglia, which has been proposed as a potential model for toxic peripheral neuropathy, have been shown to reproduce electrophysiologic and pharmacologic properties present in intact nervous tissue (Spencer et al., 1986). Organotypic cultures, once established, may be maintained in a stable state for prolonged periods. Examples given to show the promise of the approach for detecting and identifying adverse effects include the induction of structural changes in motor axons in cord-ganglion-muscle cocultures by extended contact (weeks) with n-hexane, analogous to its effects in humans and animals exposed to the solvent.

The development of practical screens for assessing CNS-specific (and/or peripheral) toxic effects involves more than mastery of the technical aspects of reproducing relative *in vivo* potency and responses. There are economic and conceptual factors, among others, that also need to be considered. One way to improve efficiency and reproducibility and reduce animal usage and costs further is to adapt assay procedures wherever possible for use in disposable plastic multiwell chambers to increase the number of explants cultured per animal needed (Spencer et al., 1986). The types and number of explants most appropriate for routine screening for CNS effects is a paramount issue. Can a comprehensive but limited set of tests be deduced and developed as a general screen for sensory, motor, or other CNS effects and maximize reduction in animal requirements, or are these kinds of systems applicable only in special cases for specific neurotoxicant classes, as in the esterase screens cited above? The same considerations apply for reaggregated tissue cultures from different brain regions, which have also been suggested as useful for studying effects of new or untested psychotherapeutic agents (Kontur et al., 1987). The data base is too limited at present to answer these important questions.

LIVER

In the 20 years since the methodology for high yield, high viability hepatocyte suspensions became available (Berry and Friend, 1969), many studies have utilized this technique. Among these are now 700-800 published studies of a toxicologic nature in freshly isolated suspensions or primary cultures of hepatocytes, mostly from rat, but including a variety of other species and humans.

Several reviews have covered the advantages and disadvantages of cellular systems in general and hepatocytes in particular for toxicity studies (Grisham, 1979; Schwarz and Greim, 1981; Klaassen and Stacey, 1982; Suolinna, 1982; Holme, 1985; Acosta et al., 1985; Guillouzo, 1986). The major disadvantage of primary cultures for toxicity and metabolism studies is an inability to maintain cytochrome P-450 associated enzymes for a day or longer in a state similar to the intact organ. Hepatocyte suspensions are better in this regard but suffer from the limitation that they retain viability for only a few hours.

The majority of toxicity studies have dealt with aspects of mechanism. The consensus is that these hepatocellular systems provide a valuable model for such investigations, as exemplified by their extensive use and opinions expressed in the above-cited reviews. While the need to assess the similarity of the responses in hepatocyte systems to those *in vivo* to justify their use has been clearly appreciated, it is somewhat surprising that a deeper and more critical analysis of this aspect is not readily available. The purpose of this section will be to review studies specifically dealing with comparisons of *in vitro* to *in vivo* data. The analysis will necessarily be limited to investigations into toxicity per se. The reader is referred to Table 1 for pertinent information in the other areas of

TABLE 1

References on Other Applications Relevant to a Comparison of In Vivo Liver with Suspensions and Primary Cultures of Hepatocytes

Application	Reference	
Biotransformation	Fry and Bridges, 1976	Croci & Williams, 1985
	Billings et al., 1977	Grant et al., 1985
	Dougherty et al., 1980	Guillouzo et al., 1985
	Sirica & Pitot, 1980	Steward et al., 1985
	Koster et al., 1981	Green et al., 1987
	Olsen & Morland, 1981	Ratanasavanh et al., 1986
	Begue et al., 1983	Grant et al., 1987
	Blaauboer et al., 1985	Jatoe et al., 1987
	Byard & Dougherty, 1985	
Genotoxicity	Strom et al., 1981	Michalopoulos et al., 1986
	Williams et al., 1982	Holme et al., 1986
	Mirsalis et al., 1982	Butterworth, 1987
	McQueen et al., 1983	Doolittle et al., 1987
	Strom et al., 1983	Rudo et al., 1987
	Holme & Soderlund, 1984	Strom et al., 1987
	Williams, 1985	
Peroxisome proliferation	Gray et al., 1983a	
	Gray et al., 1983b	
	Mitchell et al., 1984	
	Bieri et al., 1984	
	Lake et al., 1987	
Biliary dysfunction	Schwarz et al., 1977	Stacey, 1986
	Anwer et al., 1978	Gebhardt, 1986
	Gotz et al., 1980	Reichen et al., 1987
	Tarao et al. 1982	Van Dyke & Scharschmidt, 1987
	Phillips et al., 1983	Stacey, in press
	Berr et al., 1984	Stacey & Kotecka, in press
	Brook & Vore, 1984	Kukongviriyapan & Stacey,
	Ziegler & Frimmer, 1984	in press

hepatocyte usage. The references in the table are not intended to be all-inclusive and omission does not imply that a paper is inappropriate. A recently developed technique using liver slices alternatively as a model for *in vivo* hepatoxicity is reviewed elsewhere (Smith et al., in press).

Several studies have provided data on use of hepatocytes in general for determination of toxicity, but without necessarily critically relating the responses to the *in vivo* situation (Inmon et al., 1981; McQueen and Williams, 1982; Goethals et al., 1984; Sorensen and Acosta, 1985; Reinhardt and Pelli, 1986). Studies that more specifically address the matter of *in vitro/in vivo* correlation of toxic responses fall into two primary categories: (1) studies focusing on mechanisms of action of known hepatotoxicants, and (2) studies directly comparing groups of chemicals using toxicity indices. An example of the latter is release of cytoplasmic enzymes from hepatocytes *in vitro* and determination of liver enzymes in serum from treated animals as a function of relative concentration and dose.

First Category. Carbon tetrachloride is recognized as a classic hepatotoxicant. As such it is not surprising that its effects on hepatocytes *in vitro* have been extensively studied. Long and Moore (1988) provided a comprehensive comparison of toxicity in hepatocyte cultures *in vivo*, concluding that the biochemical changes were generally similar in both systems but the response was more rapid *in vitro*. Carbon tetrachloride and chloroform toxicities in mouse hepatocyte cultures were compared by Ruch et al. (1986), who found that carbon tetrachloride was the more toxic, and SKF-525 inhibited toxicity, as occurs *in vivo*. Functional changes in the Golgi apparatus, decreased protein synthesis, and potentiation of CCl₄-induced toxicity by pretreatment of the animals with alcohol and ketones have all been reproduced in rat hepatocytes (Poli et al., 1985; Paine and Hockin, 1982; Jernigan et al., 1983; Glende and Lee, 1985). Trichloroethylene reportedly potentiates CCl₄-induced lipid peroxidation and hepatotoxicity *in vivo* (Pessayre et al., 1982), and the same effect was recently found in hepatocyte suspensions (Stacey and Kefalas, unpublished data).

Some differences have been noted but these have been related to inappropriate test concentrations or methodology. Differences in the ultrastructural changes observed in hepatocytes on treatment with CCl₄ compared with the *in vivo* pattern (e.g., Stacey and Priestly 1978a,b; Stacey and Fanning, 1981) were later related to different time-course changes occurring at high toxicant concentrations (Tyson et al., 1983; Berger et al., 1986, 1987). Another anomaly from earlier studies was the inability to detect lipid peroxidation in CCl₄-exposed hepatocytes, which was subsequently related to inappropriate methodology (Stacey et al., 1982). These examples suggest caution in concluding prematurely that the *in vitro* model may be unsuitable for a particular study.

Acetaminophen is a drug which has been widely studied for its hepatotoxicity. Marked species differences in susceptibility are observed that have been reproduced *in vitro* (Moldeus, 1978; Green et al., 1984; Holme and Soderlund, 1986; Boobis et al.,

1986). Harman and Fischer (1983) found in cultured hamster hepatocytes that acetaminophen produced all the (biochemical) characteristics of the *in vivo* toxicity, and similar or equivalent effects were also reported morphologically (Walker et al., 1983). One inconsistency, however, recently reported has been that phenobarbital pretreatment protects against toxicity *in vivo* but not *in vitro* for reasons unclear (Lupo et al., 1987). Possibly the very low levels of UDP-glucuronic acid in freshly isolated hepatocytes (Croci and Williams, 1985) compared with *in vivo* contribute to this difference, in which case cultured hepatocytes might be a more suitable system overall for acetaminophen studies. Observations in mouse hepatocyte cultures, for example, show metabolite profiles consistent with the *in vivo* (Harman and McCamish, 1986).

Galactosamine is another chemical well documented for its hepatotoxicity. The mechanism is very specific, involving depletion of uridine phosphates. Tran-Thi et al. (1983) demonstrated considerable similarity between both biochemical and morphological effects of galactosamine in hepatocyte cultures and *in vivo*, including reversal by adding uridine to the medium. Toxicity was not manifest until 26 hr after addition, slower than *in vivo*, which probably explains why toxicity was not detected after just 2 hr of incubation in an earlier study (Ozturk et al., 1984). Toxicity in cultured hepatocytes isolated from galactosamine-pretreated rats was also reduced by addition of uridine or cystamine to the medium (MacDonald et al., 1987a). This study and another from this laboratory (MacDonald et al., 1987b) indicate that hepatocytes isolated after pretreatment of the animal with the test chemical exhibit the same toxic sequelae in culture as hepatocytes retained *in situ*.

Data from many other studies may be cited but only a few additional examples of *in vitro*/*in vivo* correspondence will be catalogued here. Aflatoxin B_1 has been shown to exhibit an LC50 in primary mouse hepatocyte culture 1000-fold greater than that for rat, consistent with their relative species sensitivity *in vivo* (Hanigan and Laishes, 1984). Age-related differences in allyl alcohol-induced toxicity have been reproduced in hepatocytes isolated from rats of differing ages (Rikans and Hornbrook, 1986), with hepatocytes from old rats being more sensitive than those from young rats. Blue-green algae toxicity examined in hepatocytes *in vitro* correlated well with results in the traditional mouse bioassay (Aune and Berg, 1986; Berg and Aune, 1987). Although liver toxicity was not quantitated *in vivo* by histology or by monitoring serum enzymes, the liver was deemed the primary target organ, and liver weights were clearly increased in those samples that resulted in death of the mouse and enzyme leakage *in vitro*.

Second Category. Several studies have purposely investigated groups of chemicals with a view to comparing relative toxicity *in vitro* to that *in vivo*. Twenty-three chemicals were investigated by Tyson et al. (1980). Good correspondence was found for all but two chemicals, thioacetamide and allyl alcohol, using enzyme release to assess toxicity. A follow-up study of thirty-four chemicals using both indicators for subcellular injury and enzyme release also demonstrated good agreement between *in vivo* hepatotoxicity and toxicity to hepatocyte suspensions (Story et al., 1983). In this study allyl alcohol was toxic in the *in vitro* system, whereas thioacetamide remained negative. In general, the *in vitro/in vivo* correspondence in discriminating between hepatotoxicants and nonhepatotoxicants was considered very good. In a third study, the relative hepatotoxic potentials for five haloalkanes measured in hepatocyte suspensions and *in vivo* were ranked correctly if partition coefficients were factored into the data to reconcile the differences between solvent volatility and retention in the two systems (Tyson et al., 1983). In this study, reassurance of similarity to *in vivo* was found in the inhibition of the toxicity of lower concentrations of carbon tetrachloride by SKF-525A. The correlation has been demonstrated statistically to include six additional chlorinated aliphatics (Tyson et al., in press). Other relevant work from this laboratory has been summarized (Tyson, 1987).

Six different chemicals were evaluated by Vonen and Morland (1984) for demonstrable toxicity to hepatocytes *in vitro* and compared to known *in vivo* hepatotoxic effects. The only inconsistency that the authors noted was an inability of oxytetracycline to inhibit protein synthesis *in vitro*.

Not all studies have provided a pattern of toxicity analogous to that found *in vitro*. Gottschall et al. (1983) compared a series of ortho-substituted bromobenzenes for toxicity to hepatocytes in suspension. They found poor correlation to the *in vivo* toxicity previously determined in their laboratory. A previous paper, however, reported a better correlation using somewhat different methodology (Hanzlik et al., 1982). Nevertheless such discrepancies must be satisfactorily explained and resolved to enable confidence in data from the *in vitro* systems.

Recent studies have used isolated hepatocytes to investigate mixture toxicity, and the results were compared with those *in vivo* (Stacey, 1987; Stacey et al., 1988; Stacey, in press; Stacey, submitted). As summarized in Table 2, in eight of ten mixtures tested the findings *in vitro* were consistent with *in vivo*. These initial results are promising for this application.

Another approach to use of hepatocytes *in vitro* is found in the earliest toxicological studies using this system. Zimmerman et al. (1974) used hepatocyte suspensions to investigate drugs that cause a so-called idiosyncratic hepatotoxicity in humans. They determined that erythromycin estolate, which produces jaundice, was toxic while the base and propionate, which do not, were not. Other laboratories have carried out studies using a similar rationale (Stacey et al., 1978; Dujovne and Salhab, 1980; Guillouzo et al., 1985; Oldham et al., 1985; Zimmerman et al., 1986; Boelsterli et al., 1987; Norbury et al., 1987). In these studies, it has generally been found that those drugs associated with human hepatotoxicity are clearly more cytotoxic to hepatocytes *in vitro*. While the scientific basis for these empirical observations is perhaps obscure, the consistency of the correlation does suggest the use of *in vitro* hepatocyte preparations as a screening procedure early in drug development. The situation with benoxaprofen is an interesting example in this respect; this drug was withdrawn after cases of

TABLE 2
Summary of Toxicities of Chemical Combinations to Isolated Rat Hepatocytes and to Liver

Mixture	Hepatocytes In Vitro	In Vivo
Cd + CF[a]	Yes[b]	Yes
CT + CF	Yes	Yes
CT + TE	Yes	Yes
CF + TE	Yes	No[b]
CT + CF + TE	Yes	No
Tri + Tet	Yes	Yes
Tri + TE	Yes	Yes
Tet + TE	Yes	Yes
Tri + Tet + TE	Yes	Yes
Tri + CT	Yes	Yes

[a]Abbreviations: Cd = cadmium; CF = chloroform; CT = carbon tetrachloride; TE = 1,1,1-trichloroethane; Tri = trichloroethylene; Tet = tetrachloroethylene.
[b]"Yes" means that increased toxicity was demonstrated by the combination as compared to chemicals alone. "No" means that it was not.

hepatotoxicity and other side effects were reported. Knights et al. (1986) subsequently demonstrated a clear toxicity of benoxaprofen to isolated hepatocytes.

In conclusion, there is a substantial body of evidence of similarity of response between *in vivo* hepatotoxicity and toxicity to both suspensions and primary cultures of hepatocytes. There are and will continue to be discrepancies that require resolution, and much more extensive validation for screening is still needed. Nevertheless, the overall outlook from the literature and our own experience is positive and some laboratories are even now using these systems as practical screens. One aspect that should always be remembered is that those chemicals that cause a non-organ-specific cytotoxicity will produce the same effects on hepatocytes (Zimmerman and Abernathy, 1983; Ekwall and Ekwall, 1988). If one is concerned about using *in vitro* systems to predict primary target organ effects *in vivo*, one conceivably could test both in hepatocytes (or the primary cell system of interest) and in a validated cell line to determine if the former is more sensitive and therefore more likely to be a target cell. The most important driving force for use of hepatocyte or other primary cell systems for screening is that in principle they allow the assessment of the innate, intrinsic susceptibility of that tissue to a hepatotoxicant.

KIDNEY

The development of practical isolated tubule systems for nephrotoxicity investigations and screening has lagged behind that of hepatocytes. Some reasons for this are the structural heterogeneity of the nephrons themselves, complicating the isolation procedure, the short lifetime of cells and tubular fragments in suspensions, uncertainties as to the cell type or origin when isolated cells or cell lines are used, and dedifferentiation or cell migration when freshly isolated cell or tubular fragments are attached in culture, among others. Since the cortical proximal tubule is a principal target site for chemical-induced nephropathies, most attention has focused on preparing viable isolates from these. Glomerular epithelial cell and medullary interstitial cell cultures and suspensions of tubular fragments of thick ascending limbs of Henle from the outer medulla that exhibit the appropriate target site response to selected nephrotoxicants have also been prepared (Cunarro and Weiner, 1978; Bach et al., 1986), but these will not be reviewed here. Likewise, cell lines have been developed from kidney proximal epithelial cells and used fairly extensively in nephrotoxicity studies (Handler, 1986), but, with one exception, these systems will not be critiqued for reasons given later in this section.

A variety of proximal tubule cell or fragment preparations have been developed and examined as potential nephrotoxicity screens. Smith et al. (1986) evaluated the response of mercuric chloride, cadmium chloride, and acetaminophen in a primary culture system of cortical epithelial cells from neonatal rats. Several similarities in the response pattern to *in vivo* experimental results were noted, prompting the suggestion that the culture system may have value for detecting potential nephrotoxicants. Smith et al. (1987) also studied cephaloridine-induced toxicity in these cultures using a comprehensive battery of indicators. Depression of mitochondrial succinate dehydrogenase and plasma membrane Na^+/K^+-ATPase activities were the most sensitive changes seen with the antibiotic. The relation of these changes to lipid peroxidation, which has been proposed as the mechanism of action for cephaloridine (Goldstein and Hook, 1986), was not examined.

A rank order correlation of relative nephrotoxic potentials was obtained for cephaloridine (CPH), cefazolin (CPZ), and cephalothin (CLT) by testing in rabbit proximal tubule cultures after the cells formed a confluent monolayer (Ford et al., 1986, 1988). Dye exclusion (nigrosin) was used to assess cell viability as the cytotoxic indicator. After a 48-hr incubation the ranking, in decreasing order of potency, was CLT > CPH > CPZ. Addition of rabbit kidney 9000 × *g* supernatant (KS9) to the cultures preferentially reduced CLT toxicity to obtain the proper ranking based on *in vivo* data in the rabbit. Likewise, supplementation of rabbit kidney cell line LLC-RK cultures with a KS9 fraction in a similar assay produced the same nephrotoxicity ranking for six cephalosporins as obtained *in vivo* (Table 3); without S9 cephalothin was again more toxic than anticipated (Williams et al., 1988).

The reason why KS9 incorporation into the medium corrects the toxicity ranking is

TABLE 3
In Vitro/In Vivo Data on Relative Cephalosporin Nephrotoxicity

| | In Vivo | | $(TD_{50}$ in mg/ml$)^a$ In Vitro | |
| | | | $-S9^b$ | $+S9^c$ |
Antibiotic	Dose (mg/kg)	Microscopic[a]		
Cephaloridine	125	3.5	0.03	0.24
Cephaloglycin	125	4.0	0.24	0.37
Cefazolin	500	1.5	0.51	0.66
Cefoperazone	500	1.3	0.05	0.53
Cephalothin	1,000	0.0	0.11	1.08
Ceftazidime	1,000	0.0	1.05	1.26

[a]Necrosis scored as 0, none; 1, minimal; 2, mild; 3, moderate; 4, marked. TD_{50} = toxic dose for 50% cell death in 48-hr cultures.
[b]LLC-RK$_1$ cells cultured in medium 199 + 10% fetal bovine serum.
[c]Cultures same as in footnote b to which 20% rabbit kidney S9 added.
Excerpted from Williams et al. (1988).

thought to be due to desacetylation of CLT to a less toxic metabolite by S9 esterases (Hottendorf et al., 1987). Presumably this activity is too low under the incubation conditions in the cell line and in the rabbit kidney proximal tubule cultures for the correct ranking to be obtained without manipulation of these conditions or of the data by use of correction factors. Furthermore, cultures of primary kidney cells and cell lines are different morphologically and in their functional capabilities than renal cells in the intact organ (Bellemann, 1980; Smith et al., 1987; Williams et al., 1988). Obtaining the same ranking order with S9-supplemented proximal tubule cell cultures and LLC-RK cells for the cephalosporins may be fortuitous and based on nonspecific cytotoxicity mechanisms in which the characteristic features of renal cells are not critical. This aspect is appreciated in noting that the events and mechanisms leading to cell injury *in vitro* and *in vivo* need to be elucidated (Williams et al., 1988).

The matter of the requirement of S9 in assays of this kind is further complicated by other observations. Interestingly, Ford and colleagues (1988), for example, found that they obtained the proper ranking by monitoring O_2 consumption inhibition with rabbit kidney slices directly without needing KS9 supplementation. KS9 was not required to obtain the proper ranking of three β-lactam antibiotics also tested in their culture system but was when the rabbit kidney cell line, LLC-RK, was used instead of rabbit primary cells. They suggested that their renal cell system and kidney slices can be useful models for predicting the *in vivo* nephrotoxicity of antibiotics, but the need for incorporation of S9 into the assays in some cases and not in others is a troublesome issue that needs resolution.

Suspensions of proximal tubule fragments overcome one objection to the cell culture approach because they largely retain their functional and structural properties. A limitation of these preparations, however, has been their short lifetime *in vitro* (1.5-2.0 hr in most reports) for practical results. Rylander et al. (1987) studied the response of isolated proximal tubules from rabbit kidney to cadmium chloride and dichlorovinyl cysteine using several different cytotoxicity indicators. Some loss of p-aminohippuric acid uptake capability ($\sim$ 50%) was observed during 4-hr incubations but other parameters measured were reasonably well maintained. The preparations were sufficiently useful to distinguish differences in target sites in the cells involved in the mechanisms of action of these agents, as well as for the authors to recommend them as a potential system for screening for nephrotoxins (Rylander et al., 1985). Schnellmann and Mandel (1986) found, also in rabbit kidney proximal tubule suspensions, that the rank order of potency for bromobenzene, 2-bromophenol, and 2-bromohydroquinone assessed by measuring LDH release and nystatin-stimulated and ouabain-inhibited O_2 consumption agreed well with *in vivo* data on their relative nephrotoxic potentials.

Sina et al. (1986/87) developed an *in vitro* assay for relative cytotoxicity using rabbit proximal tubule fragments attached to culture dishes. The procedure was evaluated using a series of cephalosporin and aminoglycoside antibiotics. The drug was added at the time of plating, and protein synthesis was monitored 20 hr later. The relative nephrotoxic potency of the drugs *in vitro* was based on determining D_{37} values, the concentrations at which ^{3}H-leucine incorporation into cell proteins was reduced to 37% of control values. Four of five cephalosporins exhibited the same rank order *in vitro* as *in vivo*, based on tubular necrosis seen histologically at the same administered dose; the fifth, CLT, was, as above, relatively more toxic than expected *in vitro*. When the D_{37} values for CPH, CPZ and CLT were adjusted by factoring in relative clearance times for these antibiotics, determined either in a mouse pharmacokinetic assay used by the authors or published values for the rabbit, the difference in the rankings was corrected (Table 4).

Four aminoglycosides were also tested in this system. Gentamicin, neomycin, and streptomycin D_{37} values ranged from 0.25 mM to 0.44 mM; kanamycin was less toxic with a D_{37} of 0.9 mM. The relative nephrotoxic potentials deduced from a composite of data from animal experiments and clinical observations were neomycin > gentamicin > kanamycin > streptomycin (Seale and Rennert, 1982); streptomycin and kanamycin were notably reversed in the *in vitro* studies. Definitive *in vivo* nephrotoxicity data in the rabbit were not available for validation purposes.

Recently a new method for isolating proximal tubule fragments with improved survival time in suspension and retention of energy coupled functions has been

TABLE 4
Correction of D_{37} Data by In Vivo Pharmacokinetics

Antibiotic	D_{37}[b]	$C \times T$[c]	$C \times T/D_{37}$
Using mouse *in vivo* data[a]			
Cephaloridine	0.7	5.6	8.0
Cefazolin	3.0	3.0	1.0
Cephalothin	1.75	1.0	0.6
Using rabbit *in vivo* data[d]			
Cephaloridine	0.7	12.9	18.4
Cefazolin	3.0	3.3	1.1
Cephalothin	1.75	1.0	0.6

[a]Data generated from mouse pharmacokinetic assay.
[b]D_{37} determined *in vitro* in rabbit tubule assay.
[c]Relative concentration $\times$ time for 50% clearance of the drug from the kidney.
[d]From published data.
Excerpted from Sina et al. (1986/87).

developed (Green et al., manuscript submitted). Tubule fragments were prepared by a one-step perfusion method with a buffer containing collagenase and deferoxamine, an iron chelator that inhibits lipid peroxidation. The *in vitro* viability and longevity of renal proximal tubules isolated with deferoxamine were dramatically improved compared to tubules prepared by conventional techniques (Figure 1). During long-term suspension incubation of the proximal tubule fragments, the adenine nucleotide levels, ATP/ADP ratios, and the extent of nystatin stimulation of oxygen consumption (a measure of maximum respiratory capacity) were relatively stable for up to 16 hr after an initial equilibration period. Glutathione levels and the basal rate of oxygen consumption decreased concomitantly with tubule viability, as indicated by the loss of intracellular LDH to the medium, with these parameters exhibiting less than 25% change in 8 hr. This is at least double the survival time of other preparations reported in the literature. The suitability of these preparations as a screen for renal cytotoxicants is being evaluated.

Kidney slices are often used in nephrotoxicity studies but their value as general screens has been limited by technical factors (reproducibility, uniformity, orientation) and

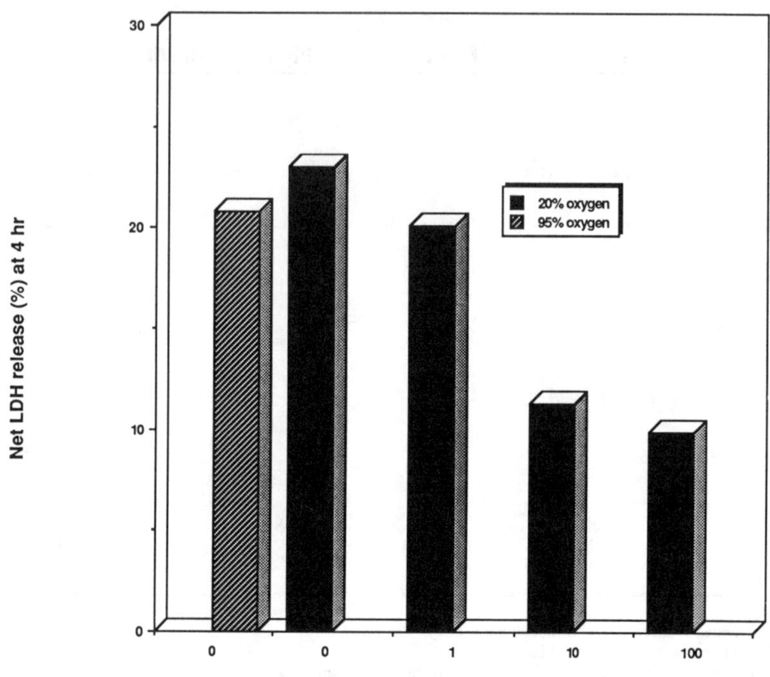

FIGURE 1.

lifetime *in vitro*. Smith (1988) recently reported that the relative degree of toxicity in this model, measured after a 2-hr preincubation exposure to the chemical followed by 1.5 hr in fresh incubation medium without test chemical, was reasonably consistent with the nephrotoxic potency *in vivo* for seven widely differing chemical entities. She did not view the model as appropriate for screening chemicals of unknown nephrotoxicity, however, considering its greatest value to be for mechanistic investigations.

Brendel and colleagues alternatively developed a slice support system for isolated rabbit kidney sections prepared by a modification of the slice method of Krumdieck et al. (1980). Functional integrity is maintained for up to 30 hr (Ruegg et al., 1987a). With cortical slices cell swelling in the apical portions occluded the tubular lumina within 2 hr, but this commonly occurs with isolated tubule suspensions as well. In some studies incubations were at room temperature and in others 0.1% penicillin was added in efforts to control bacterial contamination and growth (Ruegg et al., 1987b; Phelps et al., 1987). Besides the extended lifetime, the preparations offer a means of studying cell-specific reactions.

Ruegg et al. (1987b) used $HgCl_2$ and $K_2Cr_2O_7$ to demonstrate that the specificity of these nephrotoxicants for different segments of the proximal tubule could be reproduced in the system. Intracellular K^+ content was an early and sensitive change; histological examination has been used to confirm the injury and identify the cell types(s) involved (personal communication). Slices stressed under hypoxic conditions exhibited selective injury to the convoluted proximal tubule portion of the nephron as observed in *in vivo* clamped ischemia models. Reoxygenation after 2.25 hr, however, did not result in repair or progression of the injury to the straight proximal tubule segment, as was observed in the ischemic model. Other factors such as humoral or possibly neutrophils, a cell type implicated in reperfusion injury (Hurst, 1988), could conceivably be added to the system to generate the correct response, but these modifications may not be justified in the routine testing of chemicals for nephrotoxic potential.

Phelps et al. (1987) used precision-cut slices from rabbit cortex incubated in rotating vials for 24 hr with periodic reoxygenation to study the effects of platinum coordination complexes. Four complexes were ranked for nephrotoxic potential based on concentration times required to produce a 50% decrease in either intracellular K^+ or ATP content. The ranking obtained was found to be quite similar to clinical reports of the maximum tolerated doses for these agents. Furthermore, the concentration range for producing significant toxicity with cisplatin was in the same range or lower than peak blood levels in cancer patients and platinum uptake was comparable to *in vivo* levels. However, *in vivo* the lesion is localized in the S_3 segment whereas *in vitro* the histological changes seen were in the S_1 and S_2 segments.

One main advantage of the slice method is the much longer incubation times than has historically been possible with proximal tubule suspensions. Phelps et al. (1988) showed that 10^{-3} M cisplatin reduced slice K^+ content significantly beginning at 6 hr and the change increased dramatically at 8 and 12 hr even at low concentrations. No significant change occurred at 10^{-3} M cisplatin in LDH leakage or intracellular ATP or K^+ in proximal tubules at 6 hr. Although organic ion uptake was depressed significantly by 6 hr, control cells themselves had lost 80% or more of their original capability in this regard.

CONCLUSIONS

The survey conducted here indicates that, while the advantages of *in vitro* systems for toxicity studies have long been appreciated, progress in their development and evaluation as screens has been propelled greatly in recent years by efforts to reduce animal usage. Much more effort is needed in the areas of systems development and validation before the full potential (and limitations) of these approaches is appreciated. The results to date, although illustrating many problems that need resolution and gaps in the data and knowledge bases, are to us encouraging. The benefits for reducing animal requirements and testing costs, which have been illustrated for hepatocyte screens (Tyson, 1987), can be applied to other tissues as well. For example, with kidney proximal tubule suspensions as a test system sacrifice of one rat affords enough tissue/kidneys for 20 to 25 separate experiments in 25-ml reaction flasks (J. E. Dabbs and C. E. Green, unpublished observations) and many more if adapted for use with multiwell chambers. It may be argued that results in these systems, when validated for screening purposes, add more significance from a mechanistic standpoint as well. Furthermore, demonstrations that responses in particular *in vitro* systems correlate in detail with those in the corresponding target organs in laboratory animals for various chemicals is the first step in validating these systems for human tissues. To the extent that the latter are available and can be used for toxicity testing, use of tissues from other animal species for a number of toxicologic test needs may ultimately be eliminated altogether (Frazier et al., in press).

ACKNOWLEDGMENTS

Work reported here on kidney tubule systems development in one author's laboratory (C. Tyson) was supported in part by National Institutes of Health Contract Number ES-55109. Drs. Jay Gandolfi and Grushenka Wolfgang made useful suggestions on an earlier draft of the manuscript that were appreciated.

REFERENCES

ACOSTA, D., SORENSEN, E.M.B., ANUFORO, D.C., MITCHELL, D.B., RAMOS, K., SANTONE, K.S. and SMITH, M.A. (1985). An *in vitro* approach to the study of drugs and chemicals. In Vitro, Cell Dev. Biol. **21**:495–504.

ANWER, M.S., KROKER, R. and HEGNER, D. (1978). Inhibition of hepatic uptake of bile acids by rifamycins. Naunyn-Schmiedeberg's Arch. Pharmacol. **302**:19–24.

AUNE, T. and BERG, K. (1986). Use of freshly prepared rat hepatocytes to study toxicity of blooms of the blue-green algae Microcystis aeruginosa and Oscillatoria agardhii. J. Toxicol. Environ. Hlth. **19**:325–336.

BACH, P.H., KETLEY, C.P., AHMED, I. and DIXIT, M. (1986). The mechanisms of target cell injury by nephrotoxins. Food Chem. Toxicol. **24**:775–779.

BEGUE, J.M., BIGOT, J.F.L., GUILLOUZO, C.G., KIECHEL, J.R. and GUILLOUZO, A. (1983). Cultured human adult hepatocytes; a new model for drug metabolism studies. Biochem. Pharmacol. **32**:1643–1646.

BELLEMANN, P. (1980). Primary monolayer culture of liver parenchymal cells and kidney cortical tubules as a useful new model for biochemical pharmacology and experimental toxicology. Arch. Toxicol. **44**:63–84.

BERG, K. and AUNE, T. (1987). Freshly prepared rat hepatocytes used in screening the toxicity of blue-green algal blooms. J. Toxicol. Environ. Health **20**:187–197.

BERGER, M.L., BHATT, H., COMBES, B. and ESTABROOK, R.W. (1986). CCl_4-induced toxicity in isolated hepatocytes: the importance of direct solvent injury. Hepatology **6**:36–45.

BERGER, M.L., REYNOLDS, R.C. and COMBES, B. (1987). Carbon tetrachloride-induced morphologic alterations in isolated rat hepatocytes. Exp. Molec. Pathol. **46**:245–257.

BERR, F., SIMON, F.R. and REICHEN, J. (1984). Ethynylestradiol impairs bile salt uptake and Na-K pump function of rat hepatocytes. Am. J. Physiol. **247**:G437–443.

BIERI, F., BENTLEY, P., WAECHTER, F. and STAUBLI, W. (1984). Use of primary cultures of adult rat hepatocytes to investigate mechanisms of action of nafenopin, a hepatocarcinogenic peroxisome proliferator. Carcinogenesis **5**:1033–1039.

BILLINGS, R.E., McMAHON, R.E., ASHMORE, J. and WAGLE, S.R. (1977). The metabolism of drugs in isolated rat hepatocytes. A comparison with in vivo drug metabolism and drug metabolism in subcellular liver fractions. Drug Metab. Disp. **5**:518–525.

BLAAUBOER, B.J., VAN HOLSTEIJN I., VAN GRAFT, M. and PAINE, A.J. (1985). The concentration of cytochrome P-450 in human hepatocyte culture. Biochem. Pharmacol. **34**:2405–2408.

BOELSTERLI, U.A., BOUIS, P. and DONATSCH, P. (1987). Relative cytotoxicity of psychotropic drugs in cultured rat hepatocytes. Cell Biol. Toxicol. **3**:231–250.

BONDY, S.C. (1982). Neurotransmitter binding interactions as a screen for neurotoxicity. *In*: Mechanisms of Actions of Neurotoxic Substances. (Prasad, K.N. and Vernadakis, A., eds.), pp. 25–50, Raven Press, New York.

BOOBIS, A.R., TEE, L.B.G., HAMPDEN, C.E. and DAVIES, D.S. (1986). Freshly isolated hepatocytes as a model for studying the toxicity of paracetamol. Food Chem. Toxicol. **24**:731–736.

BRADBURY, M.W.B. (1985). The blood-brain barrier *in vitro*. Neurochem. Int. **7**:27–28.

BROCK, W. and VORE, M. (1984). The effect of pregnancy and treatment with 17B-estradiol on the transport of organic anions into isolated rat hepatocytes. Drug Metab. Dis. **12**:712–716.

BUTTERWORTH, B.E. (1987). Measurement of chemically induced DNA repair in hepatocytes *in vivo* and *in vitro* as an indicator of carcinogenic potential. *In*: The isolated hepatocyte: use in toxicology and xenobiotic biotransformation. (E.J. Rauckman and G.M. Padilla, eds.), pp. 241–264, Academic Press, New York.

BYARD, J.L. and DOUGHERTY, K.K. (1985). Comparative metabolism and toxicity of chemical carcinogens in primary cultures of hepatocytes. In Vitro **21**:489–494.

CLEMENTI, F., CABRINI, D., GOTTI, C., FORNASARI, D. and SHER, E. (1987). A human neuroblastoma cell line for neurotoxicity testing *in vitro*: effects of heavy metals. *In*: Model Systems in Neurotoxicology. Alternative Approaches to Animal Testing. (Shakar, A. and Goldberg, A.M., eds.), pp. 137–149, Alan R. Liss, Inc., New York.

CROCI, T. and WILLIAMS, G.M. (1985). Activities of several Phase I and Phase II xenobiotic biotransformation enzymes in cultured hepatocytes from male and female rats. Biochem. Pharmacol. **34**:3029–3035.

CUNARRO, J.A. and WEINER, M.W. (1978). Effects of ethacrynic acid and furosemide on respiration of isolated kidney tubules: the role of ion transport and the source of metabolic energy. J. Pharmacol. Exp. Therap. **206**:198–206.

DEWAR, A.J. (1981). Neurotoxicity testing - with particular reference to biochemical methods. *In*: Testing for Toxicity. (Gorrod, J.W., ed.), pp. 199–217, Taylor & Francis, Ltd., London.

DOOLITTLE, D.J., MULLER, G. AND SCRIBNER, H.E. (1987). The *in vivo-in vitro* hepatocyte assay for assessing DNA repair and DNA replication: Studies in the CD-1 mouse. Food Chem. Toxicol. **25**:399–405.

DOUGHERTY, K.K., SPILMAN, S.D., GREEN, C.E., STEWARD, A.R . and BYARD, J.L. (1980). Primary cultures of adult mouse and rat hepatocytes for studying the metabolism of foreign chemicals. Biochem. Pharmacol. **29**:2117–2124.

DUJOVNE, C.A. and SALHAB, A.S. (1980). Erythromycin estolate vs. erythromycin base, surface excess properties and surface scanning changes in isolated liver cell systems. Pharmacology **20**:285–291.

EKWALL, B. (1980a). Preliminary studies on the validity of *in vitro* measurement of drug toxicity using HeLa cells II. Drug toxicity in the MIT-24 system compared with mouse and human lethal dosage of 52 drugs. Toxicol. Lett. **5**:309–317.

EKWALL, B. (1980b). Screening of toxic compounds in tissue culture. Toxicology **17**:127–142.

EKWALL, B. (1980c). Toxicology to HeLa cells of 205 drugs as determined by the metabolic inhibition test supplemented by microscopy. Toxicology **17**:273–295.

EKWALL, B. and ACOSTA, D. (1982). *In vitro* comparative toxicity of selected drugs and chemicals in HeLa cells, Chang liver cells, and rat hepatocytes. Drug Chem. Toxicol. **5**:219–231.

EKWALL, B. and EKWALL, K. (1988). Comments on the use of diverse cell systems in toxicity testing. ATLA **15**:193–201.

FISHER, G.L. and PLACKE, M.E. (1987). *In Vitro* models of lung toxicity. Toxicology **47**:71–93.

FOUNTAIN, S.B. and TEYLER, T.J. (1987). Characterizing neurotoxicity using the *in vitro* hippocampal brain slice preparation: heavy metals. *In*: Model Systems in Neurotoxicology. Alternative Approaches to Animal Testing. (Shakar, A. and Goldberg, A.M., eds.), pp. 19–31, Alan R. Liss, Inc., New York.

FRAZIER, J.M., TYSON, C.A., McCARTHY, C., McCORMICK, J., MYERS, D., POWIS, G. and DUCAT, L. Potential use of human tissues for toxicity studies and testing—a minireview. Toxicol. Appl. Pharmacol. (in press).

FRY, J.R. and BRIDGES, J.W. (1976). The metabolism of xenobiotics in cell suspension and cell cultures. *In*: Prog. Drug Metab. (J.W. Bridges and Chasseaud, eds), Vol. 2, pp. 71–117. John Wiley & Son, New York.

GARDNER, D.E., CRAPO, J.D. and MASSARO, E.J. (1988). Toxicology of the lung. Raven Press, New York.

GEBHARDT, R. (1986). Use of isolated and cultured hepatocytes in studies on bile formation. *In*: Isolated and cultured hepatocytes. (A. Gullouzo and C. Guguen-Gullouzo, eds.), pp. 353–376. John Libbey Eurotext Ltd., France.

GLENDE, E.A., JR. and LEE, P.Y. (1985). Isopropanol and chlordecone potentiation of carbon tetrachloride liver injury: retention of potentiating action in hepatocyte suspensions prepared from rats given isopropanol or chlordecone. Exp. Molec. Pathol. **42**:167–174.

GOETHALS, F., KRACK, G., DEBOYSER, D., VOSSEN, P. and ROBERFROID, M. (1984). Critical biochemical function of isolated hepatocytes as sensitive indicators of chemical toxicity. Fundam. Appl. Toxicol. **4**:441–450.

GOLDSTEIN, R.S. and HOOK, J.B. (1986). Biochemical mechanisms of cephaloridine nephrotoxicity. Dev. Toxicol. Environ. Sci. **14**:41–50.

GOTTSCHALL, D.W., WILEY, R.A. and HANZLIK, R.P. (1983). Toxicity of ortho-substituted bromobenzenes to isolated hepatocytes: comparison to *in vivo* results. Toxicol. Appl. Pharmacol. **69**:55–65.

GOTZ, R., SCHWARZ, L.R. and GREIM, H. (1980). Effects of pentachlorophenol and 2,4,6-trichlorophenol on the disposition of sulfobromophthalein and respiration of isolated liver cells. Arch. Toxicol. **44**:147–155.

GRANT, M.H., BURKE, M.D., HAWKSWORTH, G.M., DUTHIE, S.J., ENGESET, J. and PETRIE, J.C. (1987). Human adult hepatocytes in primary monolayer culture. Biochem. Pharmacol. **36**:2311–2316.

GRANT, M.H., MELVIN, M.A.L., SHAW, P., MELVIN, W.T. and BURKE, M.D. (1985). Studies on the maintenance of cytochromes P-450 and b5, monooxygenases and cytochrome reductases in primary cultures of rat hepatocytes. FEBS Lett. **190**:99–103.

GRAY, T.J.B., LAKE, B.G., BEAMAND, J.A., FOSTER, J.R. and GANGOLI, S.D. (1983). Peroxisomal effects of phthalate esters in primary cultures of rat hepatocytes. Toxicology **28**:167–179.

GRAY, T.J.B. and BEAMAND, J.A. (1984). Effect of some phthalate esters and other testicular toxins on primary cultures of testicular cells. Chem. Toxicol. **22**:123–132.

GRAY, T.J.B., MOSS, E.J., CREASY, D.M. and GANGOLLI, S.D. (1985). Studies on the toxicity of some glycol esters and alkoxyacetic acids in primary testicular cell cultures. Toxicol. Appl. Pharmacol. **79**:490–501.

GREEN, C.E., DABBS, J.E., TYSON, C.A. and RAUCKMAN, E. The effect of oxygen tension and antioxidants on isolated rat renal proximal tubules. Submitted for publication.

GREEN, C.E., DABBS, J.E. and TYSON, C.A. (1984). Metabolism and cytotoxicity of acetaminophen in hepatocytes isolated from resistant and susceptible species. Toxicol. Appl. Pharmacol. **76**:139–149.

GREEN, C.E., LeVALLEY, S.E. and TYSON, C.A. (1986). Comparison of amphetamine metabolism using isolated hepatocytes from five species including human. J. Pharmacol. Exp. Ther. **237**:931–936.

GRISHAM, J.W. (1979). Use of hepatic cell cultures to detect and evaluate the mechanisms of action of toxic chemicals. Int. Rev. Exp. Pathol. **20**:123–210.

GUILLOUZO, A., BEGUE, J.M., CAMPION, J.P., GASCOIN, M.N. and GUGUEN-GUILLOUZO, C. (1985). Human hepatocyte cultures: a model of pharmacotoxicological studies. Xenobiotica **15**:635–641.

GUILLOUZO, A., BEAUNE, P., GASCOIN, M.N., BEGUE, J.M., CAMPION, J.P., GUENGERICH, F.P. and GUGUEN-GUILLOUZO, C. (1985). Maintenance of cytochrome p-450 in cultured adult human hepatocytes. Biochem. Pharmacol. **34**:2991–2995.

GUILLOUZO, A. (1986). Use of isolated and cultured hepatocytes for xenobiotic metabolism and cytotoxicity studies. *In*: Isolated and cultured hepatocytes. (A. Guillouzo and C. Guguen-Gillouzo, eds.), pp. 313–332. John Libbey Eurotext Ltd., France.

HANDLER, J.S. (1986). The use of cultured kidney cells to study renal toxicology. *In*: Nephrotoxicity of Antibiotics and Immunosuppressants. (T. Tanabe, J.B. Hook, and H. Endou, eds.), pp. 189–197, Elsevier Science Publishers, New York.

HANIGAN, H.M. and LAISHES, B.A. (1984). Toxicity of aflatoxin B1 in rat and mouse hepatocytes *in vivo* and *in vitro*. Toxicology **30**:185–193.

HANZLIK, R.P., GILLESSE, T.J. and WILEY, R.A. (1982). Toxicity and covalent binding of substituted bromobenzenes to isolated hepatocytes. Adv. Exp. Med. Biol. **136A**:381–386.

HARMAN, A.W. and FISCHER, L.J. (1983). Hamster hepatocytes in culture as a model for acetaminophen toxicity: studies with inhibitors of drug metabolism. Toxicol. Appl. Pharmacol. **71**:330–341.

HARMAN, A.W. and McCAMISH, L.E. (1986). Age-related toxicity of paracetamol in mouse hepatocytes. Biochem. Pharmacol. **35**:1731–1735.

HOLME, J.A. and SODERLUND, E.J. (1984). Unscheduled DNA synthesis of rat hepatocytes in monolayer culture. Mutat. Res. **126**:205–214.

HOLME, J.A. and SODERLUND, E. (1986). Species differences in cytotoxic and genotoxic effects of phenacetin and paracetamol in primary monolayer cultures of hepatocytes. Mutat. Res. **164**:167–175.

HOLME, J.A. (1985). Xenobiotic metabolism and toxicity in primary monolayer cultures of hepatocytes. NIPH Annals **8**:49–63.

HOLME, J.A., TRYGG, B. and SODERLUND, E. (1986). Species differences in the metabolism of 2-acetylaminofluorene by hepatocytes in primary monolayer culture. Canc. Res. **46**:1627–1632.

HOTTENDORF, G.H., LASKA, D.A., WILLIAMS, P.D. and FORD, S.M. (1987). The role of desacetylation in the detoxification of cephatholin in renal cells in culture. J. Toxicol. Environ. Health **22**:101–111.

HURST, J.K. (1988). Oxygen activation by neutrophils. *In*: Oxygen Complexes and Oxygen Activation by Transition Metals. (A. E. Martell and D. T. Sawyer, eds), pp. 149–174, Plenum Press, New York.

INMON, J., STEAD, A., WATERS, M.D. and LEWTAS, J. (1981). Development of a toxicity test system using primary rat liver cells. In Vitro **17**:1004–1010.

JATOE, S.D. and GORROD, J.W. (1987). The *in vitro*/*in vivo* comparative metabolism of 4-aminobiphenyl using isolated hepatocytes. Arch. Toxicol. **60**:65–68.

JERNIGAN, J.D., POUNDS, J.G. and HARBISON, R.D. (1983). Potentiation of chlorinated hydrocarbon toxicity by 2,5-hexanedione in primary cultures of adult rat hepatocytes. Fund. Appl. Toxicol. **3**:22–26.

JOHNSON, M.K. (1977). Improved assay of neurotoxic esterase for screening organophosphates for delayed neurotoxicity potential. Arch. Toxicol. **37**:113–115.

KLAASSEN, C.D. and STACEY, N.H. (1982). Use of isolated hepatocytes in toxicity assessment. *In*: Toxicology of the liver. (G. Plaa and W.R. Hewitt, eds.), pp. 147–179. Raven Press, New York.

KLAASSEN, C.D. (1986). Principles of toxicology. *In*: Casarett and Doull's Toxicology. The Basic Science of Poisons. (Klaassen, C.D., Amdur, M.O. and Doull, J., eds.), 3rd Ed., p. 16, Macmillan Publishing Co., New York.

KNIGHTS, K.M., CASSIDY, M.R. and DREW, R. (1986). Benoxaprofen induced toxicity in isolated rat hepatocytes. Toxicology **40**:327–339.

KONTUR, P.J., HOFFMANN, P.C. and HELLER, A. (1987). Neurotoxic effects of methamphetamine assessed in three-dimensional reaggregate tissue cultures. Dev. Brain Res. **31**:7–14.

KOSTER, H., HALSEMA, I., SCHOLTENS, E., KNIPPERS, M. and MULDER, G.J. (1981). Dose-dependent shifts in the sulfation and glucuronidation of phenolic compounds in the rat *in vivo* and in isolated hepatocytes. Biochem. Pharmacol. **30**:2569–2575.

KUKONGVIRIYAPAN, V. and STACEY, N.H. Inhibition of taurocholate transport by cyclosporin A in cultured rat hepatocytes. J. Pharmacol. Exp. Ther. (in press).

LAKE, B.G., GRAY, T.J.B., LEWIS, D.F.V., BEAMAND, J.A., HODDER, K.D., PURCHASE, R. and GANGOLLI, S.D. (1987). Structure-activity relationships for induction of peroxisomal enzyme activities by phthalate monoesters in primary rat hepatocyte cultures. Toxicol. Indust. Health 3:165–181.

LONG, R.M. and MOORE, L. (1988). Biochemical evaluation of rat hepatocyte primary cultures as a model for carbon tetrachloride hepatotoxicity: Comparative studies *in vivo* and *in vitro*. Toxicol. Appl. Pharmacol. **92**:295–306.

LOTTI, M. and JOHNSON, M.K. (1978). Neurotoxicity of organophosphorus pesticides: predictions can be based on *in vitro* studies with hen and human enzymes. Arch. Toxicol. **41**:215–221.

LUPO, S., YODIS, L.A., MICO, B.A. and RUSH, G.F. (1987). *In vivo* and *in vitro* hepatotoxicity and metabolism of acetaminophen in Syrian hamsters. Toxicology **44**:229–239.

MacDONALD, J.R., THAYER, K.J. and WHITE, C. (1987a). Inhibition of galactosamine cytotoxicity in an *in vivo/in vitro* hepatocellular toxicity model. Toxicol. Appl. Pharmacol. **89**:269–277.

MacDONALD, J.R., THAYER, K.J. and SMUCKLER, E.A. (1987b). Isolation and maintenance of monolayer hepatocytes from the livers of toxin-treated rats. Exp. Molec. Pathol. **46**:64–77.

McQUEEN, C.A. and WILLIAMS, G.M. (1982). Cytotoxicity of xenobiotics in adult rat hepatocytes in primary culture. Fundam. Appl. Toxicol. **2**:139–144.

McQUEEN, C.A., KREISER, D.M. and WILLIAMS, G.M. (1983). The hepatocyte primary culture/DNA repair assay using mouse or hamster hepatocytes. Environ. Mutag. **5**:1–8.

McQUEEN, C.A. *In Vitro* Models in Toxicology. Telford Press, Caldwell, NJ (in press).

MICHALOPOULOS, G.K., STROM, S.C. and JIRTLE, R.L. (1986). Use of hepatocytes for studies of mutagenesis and carcinogenesis. *In*: Isolated and cultured hepatocytes. (A. Guillouzo and C. Guguen-Guillouzo, eds.), pp. 333–352. John Libbey Eurotext Ltd., France.

MIRSALIS, J.C., TYSON, C.K. and BUTTERWORTH, B.E. (1982). Detection of genotoxic carcinogens in the *in vivo-in vitro* hepatocyte DNA repair assay. Environ. Mutag. **4**:553–562.

MITCHELL, A.M., BRIDGES, J.W. and ELCOMBE, C.R. (1984). Factors influencing peroxisome proliferation in cultured rat hepatocytes. Arch. Toxicol. **55**:239–246.

MOLDEUS, P. (1978). Paracetamol metabolism and toxicity in isolated hepatocytes from rat and mouse. Biochem. Pharmacol. **27**:2859–2863.

NORBURY, K.C., SANDIFER, S., CARTHAGE, P., SORENSEN, E.M.B. and ACOSTA, D. (1987). An interlaboratory study using postnatal rat hepatocytes to measure *in vitro* toxicity of known hepatotoxins. In Vitro Toxicol. **1**:193–202.

OLDHAM, H.G., NORMAN, S.J. and CHENERY, R.J. (1985). Primary cultures of adult rat hepatocytes—a model for the toxicity of histamine H2-receptor antagonists. Toxicology **36**:215–229.

OLSEN, H. and MORLAND, J. (1981). Sulfonamide acetylation in isolated rat liver cells. Acta Pharmacol. Toxicol. **49**:102–109.

OZTURK, M., LEMONNIER, F., CRESTEIL, D., SCOTTO, J. and LEMONNIER, A. (1984). Methionine metabolism and ultrastructural changes with D-galactosamine in isolated rat hepatocytes. Chem.-Biol. Interac. **51**:63–76.

PAINE, A.J. and HOCKIN, L.J. (1982). The maintenance of cytochrome P-450 in liver cell culture: recent studies on P-450 mediated mechanisms of toxicity. Toxicology **25**:41–45.

PESSAYRE, D., COBERT, B., DESCATOIRE, V., DEGOTT, C., BABANY, G., FUNCK-BRENTANO, C., DELAFORGE, M. and LARREY, D. (1982). Hepatotoxicity of trichloroethylene-carbon tetrachloride mixtures in rats: A possible consequence of potentiation by trichloroethylene of carbon tetrachloride-induced lipid peroxidation and liver lesions. Gastroenterology **83**:761–772.

PHELPS, J.S., GANDOLFI, A.J., BRENDEL, K. and DORR, R.T. (1987). Cisplatin nephrotoxicity: *in vitro* studies with precision-cut rabbit renal cortical slices. Toxicol. Appl. Pharmacol. **90**:501–512.

PHELPS, J.S., GANDOLFI, A.J. and BRENDEL, K. (1987). Cisplatinum toxicity in rabbit renal proximal tubule suspensions and precision-cut renal cortical slices. *In*: Approaches to Validation. Alternative Methods in Toxicology Series. Vol. V. (Goldberg, A.M., ed.), pp. 411–420, Mary Ann Liebert, Inc., New York.

PHILLIPS, M.J., OSHIO, C., MIYAIRI, M. and SMITH, C.R. (1983). Intrahepatic cholestasis as a canalicular motility disorder. Lab. Invest. **48**:205–211.

PLACKE, M.E. and FISHER, G.L. (1987). Adult peripheral lung organ culture—a model for respiratory tract toxicology. Toxicol. Appl. Pharmacol. **90**:284–298.

POLI, G., CHIARPOTTO, E., ALBANO, E., COTTALASSO, D., NANNI, G., MARINARI, U.M., BASSI, A.M. and DIANZANI, M.U. (1984). Carbon tetrachloride induced inhibition of hepatocyte lipoprotein secretion: functional impairment of Golgi apparatus in the early phases of such injury. Life Sci. **36**:533–539.

RATANASAVANH, D., BEAUNE, P., BAFFET, G., RISSEL, M., KREMERS, P., GUENGERICH, F.P. and GUILLOUZO, A. (1986). Immunocytochemical evidence for the maintenance of cytochrome P-450 isozymes, NADPH cytochrome c reductase and epoxide hydratase in pure and mixed primary cultures of adult human hepatocytes. Food Chem. Toxicol. **24**:577–578.

REICHEN, J., HOILIEN, C., LE, M. and JONES, R.H. (1987). Decreased uptake of taurocholate and ouabain by hepatocytes isolated from cirrhotic rat liver. Hepatology **7**:67–70.

REINHARDT, C.A. and PELLI, D.A. (1986). Screening for hepatoxicity using freshly isolated and cryopreserved rat hepatocytes. Food Chem. Toxicol. **24**:576.

RIKANS, L.E. and HORNBROOK, K.R. (1986). Isolated hepatocytes as a model for aging effects on hepatoxicity: studies with ally alcohol. Toxicol. Appl. Pharmacol. **84**:634–639.

RUCH, R.J., KLAUNIG, J.E., SCHULTZ, N.E., ASKARI, A.B., LACHER, D.A., PEREIRA, M.A. and GOLDBLATT, P.J. (1986). Mechanisms of chloroform and carbon tetrachloride toxicity in primary cultured mouse hepatocytes. Environ. Health Perspec. **69**:301–305.

RUDO, K., MEYERS, W.C., DAUTERMAN, W. and LANGENBACH, R. (1987). Comparison of human and rat hepatocyte metabolism and mutagenic activation of 2-acetylaminofluorene. Cancer Res. **47**:5861–5867.

RUEGG, C.E., GANDOLFI, A.J., NAGLE, R.B., KRUMDIECK, C.L. and BRENDEL, K. (1987a). Preparation of positional renal slices for study of cell-specific toxicity. J. Pharmacol. Meth. **17**:111–123.

RUEGG, C.E., GANDOLFI, A.J., NAGLE, R.B. and BRENDEL, K. (1987). Differential patterns of injury to the proximal tubule of renal cortical slices following *in vitro* exposure to mercuric chloride, potassium dichromate, or hypoxic conditions. Toxicol. Appl. Pharmacol. **90**:261–273.

RYLANDER, L.A ., PHELPS, J.S., GANDOLFI, A.J. and BRENDEL, K. (1987). *In vitro* nephrotoxicity: response of isolated renal tubules to cadmium chloride and dichlorovinyl cysteine. *In Vitro* Toxicol. **1**:111–127.

RYLANDER, L.A., GANDOLFI, A.J. and BRENDEL, K. (1985). Inhibition or organic acid/base transport in isolated rabbit renal tubules by nephrotoxins. *In: In vitro* Toxicology, Vol. 3, "Alternative Methods in Toxicology," (Goldberg, A.M., ed.), pp. 237–247, Mary Ann Liebert, Inc., New York.

SCHNELLMANN, R.G. and MANDEL, L.J. (1986). Cellular toxicity of bromobenzene and bromobenzene metabolites to rabbit proximal tubules: the role and mechanism of 2-bromohydroquinone. J. Pharmacol. Exp. Therap. **237**:456–461.

SCHWARZ, L.R. and GREIM, H. (1981). Frontiers in liver disease. *In*: Isolated hepatocytes: an analytical tool in hepatotoxicology. (P.D. Berk and T.C. Chalmers, eds.), pp. 61–79. Thieme-Stratton, New York.

SCHWARZ, L.R., SCHWENK, M., PFAFF, E. and GREIM, H. (1977). Cholestatic steroid hormones inhibit taurocholate uptake into isolated rat hepatocytes. Biochem. Pharmacol. **26**:2433–2437.

SEALE, T.W. and RENNERT, O.M. (1982). Mechanisms of antibiotic-induced nephrotoxicity. Ann. Clin. Lab. Sci. **12**:1–10.

SHAKAR, A. and GOLDBERG, A.M., eds. (1987). Model Systems in Neurotoxicology. Alternative Approaches to Animal Testing. Alan R. Liss, Inc., New York.

SINA, J.F., BEAN, C.L., BLAND, J.A., MacDONALD, J.S., NOBLE, C., ROBERTSON, R.T. and BRADLEY, M.O. (1986/87). An *in vitro* assay for cytotoxicity to proximal tubule suspensions from rabbit kidney. *In Vitro* Toxicol. **1**:13–22.

SIRICA, A.E. and PITOT, H.C. (1980). Drug metabolism and effects of carcinogens in cultured hepatic cells. Pharmacol. Rev. **31**:205–228.

SMITH, J.H. (1988). The use of renal cortical slices from the Fischer 344 rat as an *in vitro* model to evaluate nephrotoxicity. Toxicol. Appl. Pharmacol. **11**:132–142.

SMITH, M.A., ACOSTA, D. and BRUCKNER, J.V. (1986). Development of a primary culture system of rat kidney cortical cells to evaluate the nephrotoxicity of xenobiotics. Food Chem. Toxic. **24**:551–556.

SMITH, M.A., ACOSTA, D. and BRUCKNER, J.V. (1987). Cephaloridine toxicity in primary cultures of rat renal cortical epithelial cells. Toxic. *In Vitro* **1**:23–29.

SMITH, P.F., FISHER, R., McKEE, R., GANDOLFI, A.J., KRUMIDECK, C.L. and BRENDEL, K. Precision cut liver slices: a new *in vitro* tool in toxicology. *In: In vitro* Models in Toxicology. (McQueen, C.A., ed.), Telford Press, Caldwell, NJ (in press).

SMITH, R.A., ORR, D.J. and McINNES, I.B. (1987). A refined primary culture system of adult mouse sensory neurons for neurotoxicity. *In*: Model Systems in Neurotoxicology. Alternative Approaches to Animal Testing. (Shakar, A. and Goldberg, A.M., eds.), pp. 69–75, Alan R. Liss, Inc., New York.

SORENSEN, E.M.B. and ACOSTA, D. (1985). Relative toxicities of several nonsteroidal antiinflammatory compounds in primary cultures of rat hepatocytes. J. Toxicol. Environ. Health **16**:425–440.

SPENCER, P.S., CRAIN, S.M., BORNSTEIN, M.B., PETERSON, E.R. and VAN DE WATER, T. (1986). Chemical neurotoxicity: detection and analysis in organotypic cultures of sensory and motor systems. Food Chem. Toxicol. **24**:539–544.

STACEY, N.H. (1986). Effects of ethinyl estradiol on substrate uptake and efflux by isolated rat hepatocytes. Biochem. Pharmacol. **35**:2495–2500.

STACEY, N.H. (1987). Assessment of the toxicity of chemical mixtures with isolated rat hepatocytes: cadmium and chloroform. Fund. Appl. Toxicol. **9**:616–622.

STACEY, N.H. (in press). Toxicity of combinations of chlorinated aliphatic hydrocarbons *in vitro* and *in vivo*. Toxicol. *In Vitro*.

STACEY, N.H. (submitted). Toxicity of mixtures of trichloroethylene, tetrachloroethylene and 1,1,1-trichloroethane: similarity of *in vitro* to *in vivo* responses.

STACEY, N.H. Effects of chlorpromazine on taurocholate transport in isolated rat hepatocytes. Biochem. Pharmacol. (in press).

STACEY, N.H. and FANNING, J.C. (1981). Ultrastructural changes in isolated rat hepatocytes after incubation with carbon tetrachloride. Toxicology **22**:69–77.

STACEY, N.H. and KOTECKA, B. Inhibition of taurocholate and ouabain transport in isolated rat hepatocytes by cyclosporin A. Gastroenterology (in press).

STACEY, N.H., MULLER, L. and KEFALAS V. (1988). Toxicity of cadmium/chloroform combination *in vivo*. Med. Sci. Res. (in press).

STACEY, N.H., OTTENWALDER, H. and KAPPUS, H. (1982). CCl_4-induced lipid peroxidation in isolated rat hepatocytes with different oxygen concentrations. Toxicol. Appl. Pharmacol. **62**:421–427.

STACEY, N.H. and PRIESTLY, B.G. (1978a). Dose dependent toxicity of CCl_4 in isolated rat hepatocytes and the effects of hepatoprotective treatments. Toxicol. Appl. Pharmacol. **45**:29–39.

STACEY, N.H. and PRIESTLY, B.G. (1978b). Lipid peroxidation in isolated rat hepatocytes. Relationship to toxicity of CCl_4, ADP/Fe^{3+} and diethylmaleate. Toxicol. Appl. Pharmacol. **45**:41–48.

STACEY, N.H., PRIESTLY, B.G. and HALL, R.C. (1978). Toxicity of halogenated volatile anesthetics in isolated rat hepatocytes. Anesthesiology **48**:17–22.

STEWARD, A.R., DANNAN, G.A., GUZELIAN, P.S. and GUENGERICH, F.P. (1985). Changes in the concentration of seven forms of cytochrome P-450 in primary cultures of adult rat hepatocytes. Molec. Pharmacol. **27**:125–132.

STORY, D.L., GEE, S.J. and TYSON, C.A. (1983). Response of isolated hepatocytes to organic and inorganic cytotoxins. J. Toxicol. Environ. Hlth. **11**:483–501.

STROM, S., KILGERMAN, A.D. and MICHALOPOULOS, G. (1981). Comparisons of the effects of chemical carcinogens in mixed cultures of rat hepatocytes and human fibroblasts. Carcinogenesis **2**:709–715.

STROM, S.C., JIRTLE, R.L. and MICHALOPOULOS, G. (1983). Genotoxic effects of 2-acetylaminofluorene on rat and human hepatocytes. Environ. Health Perspec. **49**: 165–170.

STROM, S.C., MONTEITH, D.K., MANOHARAN, K. and NOVOTNY, A. (1987). Genotoxicity studies with human hepatocytes. *In*: The isolated hepatocyte. Use in toxicology and xenobiotic biotransformations. (E.J. Rauckman and G.M. Padilla, eds.), pp. 265–280. Academic Press, New York.

SUOLINNA, E.M. (1982). Isolation and culture of liver cells and their use in the biochemical research of xenobiotics. Med. Biol. **60**:237–254.

TARAO, K., OLINGER, E.J., OSTROW, J.D. and BALISTRERI, W.F. (1982). Impaired bile acid efflux from hepatocytes isolated from the liver of rats with cholestasis. Am. J. Physiol. **243**:G253–258.

TRAN-THI, T.A., PHILLIPS, J., FALK, H. and DECKER, K. (1985). Toxicity of D-galactosamine for rat hepatocytes in monolayer culture. Exp. Mol. Pathol. **42**:89–116.

TYSON, C.A., MITOMA, C., and KALIVODA, J. (1980). Evaluation of hepatocytes isolated by a nonperfusion technique in a prescreen for cytotoxicity. J. Toxicol. Environm. Hlth. **6**:197–205.

TYSON, C.A., HAWK-PRATHER, C., STORY, D.L. and GOULD, D.H. (1983). Correlations of *in vitro* and *in vivo* hepatotoxicity for five haloalkanes. Toxicol. Appl. Pharmacol. **70**:289–302.

TYSON, C.A., STORY, D.L. and STEPHENS, R.J. (1983). Ultrastructural changes in isolated rat hepatocytes exposed to different CC14 concentrations. Biochem. Biophys. Res. Commun. **114**:511–517.

TYSON, C.A. (1987). Correspondence of results from hepatocyte studies with *in vivo* response. Toxicol. Indus. Health **3**:459–477.

TYSON, C.A., GEE, S.J., HAWK-PRATHER, K., STORY, D.L. and MILMAN, H.A. Correlation between *in vivo/in vitro* toxicity with chlorinated aliphatics. Toxicol. *In Vitro* (in press).

VAN DYKE, R.W. and SCHARSCHMIDT, B.F. (1987). Effects of chlorpromazine on Na+–K+–ATPase pumping and solute transport in rat hepatocytes. Am. J. Physiol. **253**:G613–621.

VOLPE, L.S., BIAGIONI, T.M. and MARQUIS, J.K. (1985). *In vitro* modulation of bovine caudate muscarinic receptor number by organophosphates and carbamates. Toxicol. Appl. Pharmacol. **78**:226–234.

VONEN, B. and MORLAND, J. (1984). Isolated rat hepatocytes in suspension: potential hepatotoxic effects of six different drugs. Arch. Toxicol. **56**:33–37.

WALKER, R.M., McELLIGOTT, T.F., MASSEY, T.E. and RACZ, W.J. (1983). Ultrastructural effects of acetaminophen in isolated mouse hepatocytes. Exp. Molec. Pathol. **39**:163–175.

WHETSELL, W.O., Jr. and SCHWARZ, R. (1984). Mechanisms of excitotoxins in organotypic cultures of rat central nervous system. Wenner-Gren Cent. Int. Symp. Ser. **39**:207–219.

WILLIAMS, P.D., LASKA, D.A., TAY, L.K. and HOTTENDORF, G.H. (1988). Comparative toxicities of cephalosporin antibiotics in a rabbit kidney cell line (LLC-RK₁). Antimicrob. Agents Chemother. **32**:314–318.

WILLIAMS, G.M., LASPIA, M.F. and DUNKEL, V.C. (1982). Reliability of the hepatocyte primary culture/DNA repair test in testing of coded carcinogens and noncarcinogens. Mutat. Res. **97**:359–370.

WILLIAMS, G.M. (1985). Identification of genotoxic and epigenetic carcinogens in liver culture systems. Regul. Toxicol. Pharmacol. **5**:132–144.

ZIEGLER, K. and FRIMMER, M. (1984). Cyclosporin A protects liver cells against phalloidin. Potent inhibition of the inward transport of cholate and phallotoxins. Biochim. Biophys. Acta. **805**:174–180.

ZIMMERMAN, H.J., KENDLER, J., LIBBER, S. and LUKACS, L. (1974). Hepatocyte suspensions as a model for demonstration of drug hepatotoxicity. Biochem. Pharmacol. **23**:2187–2189.

ZIMMERMAN, H.J. and ABERNATHY, C.O. (1985). Employment of *in vivo* models for study of drug hepatotoxicity: applications of phenothiazines, related compounds, and erythromycins. *In*: Hepatology (Brunner, H. and Thaler, H., eds.), pp. 61–74. Raven Press, NY.

ZIMMERMAN, H.J., JACOB, L., BASSAN, H., GILLESPIE, J., LUKACS, L. and ABERNATHY, C.O. (1986). Effects of H2-blocking agents on hepatocytes *in vitro*: correlation with potential for causing hepatic disease in patients (42373). Proc. Soc. Exp. Biol. Med. **182**:511–14.

ACUTE OCULAR IRRITATION EVALUATION: *IN VIVO* AND *IN VITRO* ALTERNATIVES AND MAKING THEM THE "STANDARD" FOR TESTING

SHAYNE C. GAD

G.D. Searle and Co.
Skokie, Illinois

Testing for potential to cause irritation or damage to the eyes is the most active area for the development of alternatives and the most sensitive area of animal testing in biomedical research. This paper reviews available toxicology information sources. It gives a history of eye testing and objectives behind data generation and utilization. It summarizes the procedures for and the adequacy of in vivo test methods, and reviews criteria for evaluating the most important of the 60 in vitro tests now in use or under development. It argues the need for a collaborative interlaboratory validation of candidate in vitro alternative tests.

INTRODUCTION

The test methods designed and used to evaluate the potential of a man-made material to cause irritation or damage to the eye by a splash or other accidental occurrence hold a unique and ambivalent place in our society. On one hand, the eyes represent a uniquely valuable and vulnerable asset to people; the sense of vision is critical for functioning in our world, and the responsible organs are delicate and relatively unprotected. At the same time, the traditional tests (with their misuse and misunderstanding of their use) have served as the rallying point for those concerned about the humane and proper use of animals. This has caused the field of testing for potential to cause irritation or damage to the eyes to become both the most active area for the development of alternatives and innovations and the most sensitive area of animal testing and use in research.

1.   Address correspondence to: Shayne C. Gad, Ph.D., D.A.B.T., Director of Toxicology, G.D. Searle and Co., Skokie, Illinois 60077.
2.   Key words: alternative methodology, Draize test, ocular irritation.
3.   Abbreviations: ASTM, American Society for Testing and Materials; FHSA, Federal Hazardous Substances Act; HSDB, Hazardous Substances Data Bank; NIOSH, National Institute of Occupational Safety and Health; NLM, National Library of Medicine; NTP, National Toxicology Program; OTA, Office of Toxicology Assessment; PFII, Primary Dermal Irritation Index; RTECS, Registry of Toxic Effects of Chemical Substances; TDB, Toxicology Data Bank.

Tremendous progress has been made in the area of eye irritation testing. Multiple modifications and improvements to *in vivo* testing procedures now give us tests which (1) are more reliable, reproducible and predictive of potential hazards in humans, (2) use fewer animals, (3) are considerably more humane than earlier test forms. At the same time, a multitude of *in vitro* test systems have been proposed, developed, and validated to at least some extent. Yet the perception is that little has changed. Why?

It is hoped that this volume will serve to make more people aware of the new techniques which are available. But more importantly that the whole process involved in testing can be modified so that only what needs to be done will be and that such tests will answer the desired questions in as humane a manner as possible.

OBJECTIVES BEHIND IT ALL: WHY TEST?

The product safety assessment process, in the broadest sense, is a multistep process in which none of the individual steps is overwhelmingly complex, but the integration of the entire process involves fitting together a large number of pieces. This volume as a whole seeks to address the question of alternative ways of assessing the toxicology associated with agents that interact with the eyes - that is, the ocular route of exposure. How the data generated by the various test systems and models described elsewhere in this volume are used by government and private enterprise to provide for a safe product life cycle must be considered first, before any critical assessment of how testing is done. As will be seen, this is a special case of the general product safety assessment problem, and it will be addressed by starting with the general case and progressing to the special case. Along the way, limitations of current models and places where testing and research data could be made more practically useful will be pointed out.

The single most important part of a product safety evaluation program is, in fact, the initial overall process of defining and developing an adequate data package on the potential hazards associated with the product life cycle (Gad, 1988) (the manufacture, sale, use and disposal of a product and associated process materials). To do this, one must ask a series of questions in a very interactive process, with many of the questions designed to identify and/or modify their successors. The first is - what information is needed?

This calls for understanding the way in which a product is to be made and used, and the potential health and safety risks associated with exposure of humans who will be associated with these processes. This is the basis of a hazard and toxicity profile. Once such a profile is established, the available literature is searched to determine what is already known.

Taking into consideration this literature information and the previously defined exposure potential, plus such labeling requirements that might apply, a tier type approach is used to generate a list of tests which need to be done. What goes into a tier system is determined by both regulatory requirements imposed by government agencies and the philosophy of the parent organization. How such tests are actually performed is determined on one of two bases. The first (and most common) is the menu approach: selecting a series of standard design tests as "modules" of data, of which an eye irritation test or screen is one. The second, which I support, is an alternative approach, where studies are designed (or designs are selected) based both on needs and what has been learned about the product.

The initial and most important aspect of a product safety evaluation program is the series of steps that leads to an actual statement of problems or of the objectives of any testing and research program. This definition of objectives is essential and. as proposed here, consists of five steps: (1) defining product or material use, (2) quantitating or estimating exposure potential, (3) identifying potential hazards, (4) gathering baseline data, and (5) designing and defining the actual research program. Later, we will look at the specific application of this to dermal and ocular toxicity cases, where the concept of *communities of interest* will become essential.

Product/Material Use. Identifying how a material is to be used, what it is to be used for, and how it is to be made are the essential first three questions to be answered before a meaningful assessment program can be performed (Jayjock and Gad, 1988). These determine, to a large extent, how many people are potentially exposed, to what extent and by what routes they are exposed, and what benefits they perceive or gain from a product use. The answers to these questions are generally categorical or qualitative, and become quantitative (as will be reviewed in the next section) at a later step (frequently long after acute data have been generated).

Starting with an examination of how a material is to be made (or how it is already being made), it generally occurs that there are several process segments, each representing separate problems. Commonly, much of a manufacturing process is "closed" (that is, it occurs in sealed airtight systems) thereby limiting exposures to (1) leaks, and (2) maintenance and repair work. Smaller segments of the process will almost invariably not be closed. These segments are most common either where some form of manual manipulation is required, or where the segment requires a large volume of space (such as when fibers or other objects are spun, formed, or individually coated with something) or where the products is packaged (such as powders being put into bags or polymers being removed from molds). The exact manner and quantity of each segment of the manufacturing process, given the development of a categorization of exposures for each of these segments, will then serve to help quantitate the identified categories.

Likewise, consideration of what a product is to be used for and how it is to be used should help identify who, outside of the manufacturing process, may be exposed, by what routes, and to what extent.

The answers to these questions, again, will generate a categorical set of answers, but will also serve to identify which particular aspects of regulatory toxicity testing may be operative (such as those for the Department of Transportation or Consumer Products Safety Commission). If a product is to be worn (such as clothing or jewelry) or used on an environmental surface (such as household carpeting or wall covering), the potential for the exposure of a large number of people (albeit at low levels in the case of most materials) is large. If the product is to be used on exterior portions of buildings, the potential for exposure to a large number of individuals would be smaller. Likewise, the nature of the intended use (say, as a true consumer product versus an industrial product) determines the potential for extent and degree of exposure in overt and subtle manners. Likewise, in general, true consumer products (such as household cleaners) have a greater potential for both accidental exposure and misuse.

Exposure Potential. The next problem (or step) is quantitating the exposure of the human population, both in terms of how many people are exposed, by what routes (or means) and what quantities of an agent they are exposed to. For ocular testing, this is an easier problem than for dermal, oral or inhalation.

This process of identifying and quantitating exposure groups within the human population is beyond the scope of this chapter, except for some key points. Classification methods are the key tools, however, for identifying and properly delimiting human populations at risk and will be briefly discussed.

Classification is both a basic concept and a collection of techniques which are necessary prerequisites for further analysis of data when the members of a set of data are (or can be) each described by several variables (Jayjock and Gad, 1988; Glass, 1975; Gordon, 1981). At least some degree of classification (which is broadly defined as the dividing of the members of a group into smaller groups in accordance with a set of decision rules) is necessary prior to any data collection. Whether formally or informally, an investigator has to decide which things are similar enough to be counted as the same and to develop rules governing collection procedures. Such rules can be as simple as "measure and record exposures only of production workers," or as complex as that demonstrated by the expanded classification presented below. Such a classification also demonstrates that the selection of which variables to measure will determine the final classification of data.

AVAILABLE TOXICOLOGY INFORMATION
SOURCES AND THEIR USE

Sources

1. Published information sources
2. On-line literature searches
3. Colleagues
4. Monitoring published literature and other research in progress

Also to be considered is maintenance of a database once it is established (in many places this is called product surveillance).

However, before review of the literature is initiated, it is important to obtain as much of the following product composition and exposure information as practical:

1. Chemical composition and major impurities
2. Chemical production and use information, i.e., manufacturing process, exposure patterns and other commercial uses
3. Correct chemical identity including formula, Chemical Abstract Service (CAS) Number, common synonyms and trade names
4. Selected physical properties, i.e., physical state, vapor pressure, chemical reactivity and pH
5. Other chemical substances exhibiting similar toxicity and/or structure/ activity relationships

Collection of the aforementioned information is not only important for the hazard assessment (high vapor pressure would indicate high exposure potential to the material as a gas, just as high or low pH would indicate high irritation potential), but prior identification of all product uses and exposure patterns can identify alternative information sources, e.g., chemicals formerly used as anesthetics, food additives or pesticides may have extensive toxicology data obtainable from government or private sources.

Published Information Sources. There are numerous published texts for use in literature reviewing. An alphabetical listing of the more common available texts with ocular data is provided in Table 1. Obviously, this is not a complete listing and consists of only the general multipurpose texts that have a wider range of applicability for the dermal and ocular toxicity of commercial products (current or potential). Texts dealing with specialized classes of chemicals, e.g., petroleum hydrocarbons, plastics or those with specific target organ toxicities (neurotoxins and teratogens), are not considered to be within the scope of this section and the interested reader is referred to Parker (1987) or Wexler (1987) for further details.

1. Which groups are potentially exposed?
2. What are segments of groups? Consumers, production workers,neonatal patients, etc.
3. What are routes of potential exposure?
4. Which group does each route occur in?
5. Which sex is exposed?
6. Which age groups are potentially exposed?

Data classification serves two purposes: data simplification (also called a descriptive function) and prediction. Simplification is necessary because there is a limit to both the volume and complexity of data that the human mind can comprehend and deal with conceptually. Classification allows us to attach a label (or name) to each group of data, to summarize the data (that is, assign individual elements of data to groups and to characterize the population of the group), and to define the relationships between groups (that is, develop a taxonomy).

Prediction is the use of summaries of data and knowledge of the relationships between groups to develop hypotheses as to what will happen when further data are collected (as when more production or market segments are expanded) and as to the mechanisms which cause such relationships to develop. Indeed, classification is the prime device for the discovery of mechanisms in all of science. A classic example of this was Darwin's realization that there were reasons (the mechanisms of evolution) behind the differences and similarities in species which had helped Linaeus to earlier develop his initial modern classification scheme (for taxonomy) for animals.

An investigator must first understand the process involved in making, shipping, using, and disposing of a material. The Environmental Protection Agency (EPA, 1986) recently proposed guidelines for such identification and exposure quantitation. The exposure groups may be very large or relatively small populations, each with a markedly different potential for exposure differences (such as repeated exposure in humid climate) and special characteristics which contribute to or modify the hazards of exposure (such as wearing contact lenses).

Potential Hazard. Once the types of exposure have been identified and the quantities approximated, a toxicity matrix can be developed by identifying the potential hazards. Such an identification can proceed by one of the three major approaches:

1. Analogy from data reported in the literature
2. Structure-activity relationships
3. Predictive testing

TABLE 1
Published Information Sources for Dermal
and Ocular Toxicology Data

Title	Reference
Chemical Hazards of the Workplace	Proctor and Hughes, 1978
Clinical Toxicology of Commercial Products	Gosselin, et al., 1984
Criteria Documents	NIOSH
Current Intelligence Bulletins (NIOSH)	NIOSH
Dangerous Properties of Industrial Materials	Sax, 1985
Documentation of the Threshold Limit Values (AIHA)	ACGIH, 1986
Handbook of Toxic and Hazardous Chemicals	Sittig, 1986
Hygienic Guide Series (AIHA)	AIHA, 1980
Industrial Toxicology	Finkel, 1983
Merck Index	Windholz, 1983
Occupational Health Guidelines for Chemical Hazards (HIOSH/OSHA)	Mackinson, 1981
Patty's Industrial Hygiene and Toxicology	Clayton and Clayton, 1981
Physician's Desk Reference	Barnhart, 1987
Registry of Toxic Effects of Chemical Substances (RETECS)	NIOSH, 1984
Toxicology of the Eye	Grant, 1974

On-Line Literature Searches. In the last ten years, the use of on-line literature searches by many toxicologists has changed from an occasional, sporadic request to the semi-continuous need for computerized search capabilities. Usually non-toxicology related search capabilities are already in place in many companies. Therefore, all that is needed is to expand the information source to include some of the databases that cover the types of toxicology information needed. A university or a private contract laboratory can often provide this service. Most of the databases of interest to toxicologists are parts of the National Library of Medicine (NLM) system.

The NLM information retrieval service (NLM) contains Medline, Toxline and Cancerline databases. Databases commonly used by industrial toxicologists in the NLM service are briefly discussed below.

1. Toxline (Toxicology Information Online) is a bibliographic database covering the pharmacological, biochemical, physiological, environmental and toxicological effects of drugs and other chemicals. It contains approximately 1.7 million citations, most of which are complete with abstract, index terms and Chemical Abstracts Service (CAS) Registry Numbers.

2. Medline (Medical Information Online) is a database containing approximately 800,000 references to biomedical journal articles published since 1980. These articles, usually with an English abstract, are from over 3,000 journals. Coverage of previous years (back to 1966) is provided by back files, searchable online, that total some 3.5 million references.

3. Toxnet (Toxicology Data Network) is a computerized network of toxicologically oriented data banks. Toxnet offers a sophisticated search and retrieval package which accesses the following two subfiles:

    a. Hazardous Substances Data Bank (HSDB) is a scientifically reviewed and edited data bank containing toxicological information strengthened with additional data related to the environment, emergency situations, and regulatory issues. Data are derived from a variety of sources including government documents and special reports. This database contains records for over 4,100 chemical substances.

    b. Toxicology Data Bank (TDB) is a peer-reviewed data bank focusing upon toxicological and pharmacological data, environmental and occupational information, manufacturing and use data and chemical and physical properties. References have been extracted from a selective list of standard source documents.

4. Registry of Toxic Effect of Chemical Substances (RTECS) is the NLM online version of NIOSH's annual compilation of substances with toxic activity (Barnhard, 1987). The original collection of data was derived from the 1971 Toxic Substances Lists. The RTECS data contain threshold limit values, aquatic toxicity ratings, air standards, National Toxicology Program (NTP) carcinogenesis bioassay information and toxicological/carcinogenic review information. The National Institute of Occupational Safety and Health (NIOSH) is responsible for the file content in RTECS, and for providing quarterly updates to NLM. Currently, RTECS covers toxicity data on more than 61,000 substances. Greater detail on available data sources and their use in toxicology can be found in Wexler (1987) or Parker (1988).

The next step, given that no data are found from any of these sources, is to perform appropriate tests. The bulk of this volume addresses specifics of performing such tests. How did we come to the current stage in employing such tests?

HISTORY OF EYE TESTING

Early in 1930's, an untested eyelash dye containing p-phenylenediamine ("Lash Lure") was brought onto the marked in the United States. This product (as well as a number of similar products) rapidly demonstrated that it could sensitize the external ocular structures, leading to corneal ulceration with loss of vision and at least one fatality (McCally et al., 1933). This occurrence led to the revision of the Food and Drug Act, which became the Food, Drug and Cosmetic Act of 1938. To meet the provisions of this act, a number of test methods were proposed. Latven and Molitor (1939) and Mann and Pullinger (1942) were among those to first report the use of rabbits as a test model to predict eye irritation in humans. No specific scoring system, however, was presented to grade or summarize the results in these tests, and the use of animals with pigmented eyes (as opposed to albinos) was advocated. Early in 1944, Friedenwald et al. (1944) published a method that used albino rabbits in a similar manner to that of the original Draize (1944) publication, but still prescribed the description of the individual animal responses as the means of evaluating the reporting the results. Although a scoring method was provided, no overall score was generated for the test group. Draize (head of the Dermal and Ocular Toxicity Branch at the Food and Drug Administration) modified Friedenwald's procedure and made the significant addition of a summary scoring system.

Over the 40 years since the publication of the Draize scoring system, it has become common practice to call all acute eye irritation tests performed in rabbits "the Draize eye test." However, since 1944, ocular irritation testing in rabbits has significantly changed. Clearly, there is no longer a single test design that is used, and there are different objectives that are pursued by different groups using the same test.

OBJECTIVES BEHIND DATA GENERATION
AND UTILIZATION

To understand how ocular toxicity data are used, and how the data generation process might be changed to better meet the product safety assessment need, it is essential to understand that different commercial organizations have different answers to these questions. The ultimate answer is a multidimensional matrix, with the three major dimensions of the matrix (1) the toxicity data type (lethality, sensitization, corrosion, irritation, photosensitization, phototoxicity, etc.), (2) exposure characteristics (extent, population size, population characteristics, etc.), and (3) type of commercial organization (community of interest). Communities of interest are really defined by how the products are to be used, who regulates their use, and what benefits are expected for the consumer. There are a number of ways of classifying such communities, but for our purposes we will divide and define them as follows.

Pharmaceuticals: Materials of concern are agents intended as therapeutics (or medical devices) where patients or health care provider (doctor, nurse or pharmacist) has a significant chance of ocular or dermal exposures - particularly if the intended primary route of administration is ocular or topical. The Food and Drug Administration (FDA) is the United States (US) regulator.

Cosmetics and Toiletries: The materials are cosmetics, fragrances, shampoo, hand and body soaps, hair dyes and other materials intended to improve appearance and personal presentation. These are intended either to be applied to the skin and proximity of the eye, or to be applied or used in a manner that makes dermal or ocular exposure unavailable. The major US regulators are the Food and Drug Administration and Consumer Product Safety Commission.

Consumer Products: Products intended to be used by the average person in and around their home can be divided into those that have a high potential for exposure (dish and laundry detergents, for example, those that have low potential for such exposure (drain cleaners, oven cleaners, etc.), or those that have a wide range in between (such as window and carpet cleaners). The primary regulators are CPSC and DOT, but EPA also is important in terms of new chemical entities and disposal and waste management.

Agricultural Products: These products are pesticides, herbicides, fertilizers (which represent a special case), and other intentional food additives (such as preservatives, sterilants, etc.). The extent of dermal and ocular exposure will vary widely in use. Note that these could be subdivided into those agents used in the field (that is, actually used in agriculture) and those agents used in the storage and processing of foods. Ocular and dermal concerns for the former fall primarily to the EPA (under the Federal Insecticides, Fungicide and Rodenticide Act-FIFRA), with secondary considerations by DOT and FDA. The second group has FDA as the primary driving force, with EPA and DOT concerns secondary.

Industrial Chemicals: These are materials to which the major exposure is to workers involved in the manufacture and transportation of products. In a sense, all the materials (e.g., the above categories) fall into this group at some time, plus a number of other chemicals that never appear (as such) in those categories (such as hydrofluoric acid and plasticizers). These are handled by a smaller population (relative to most other products). Eye and skin contact is never intended; in fact, active measures are taken to prevent it. The use of eye and skin data in these cases is to fulfill labeling requirements for shipping and to provide hazard assessment information for accidental exposures and their treatment. The results of such tests do not directly affect the economic future of a material.

Each of these communities has different needs and uses for each of the kinds of data produced and these must be examined independently. Next, we will examine each test (endpoint case), develop a decision matrix for that type of data, and then point out the shortfalls in existing test systems.

OCULAR IRRITATION

For the pharmaceutical industry (with the exception of contact lenses, which will not be discussed here), eye irritation testing is done when the material is intended to be put into the eye as a means or route of application or for ocular therapy. There are a number of special tests applicable to pharmaceutical or medical devices that are beyond the scope of this volume, as they are not intended to assess potential acute effects or irritation. In general, however, an eye irritation test that is used by this group must be both sensitive and accurate in predicting the potential to cause irritation in humans. Failing to identify human ocular irritants (lack of sensitivity) is to be avoided, but of equal concern is the occurrence of false positives.

The cosmetics and toiletries industry is similar to the pharmaceutical industry in that the materials of interest are frequently intended for repeated application in the area of the eye. In such uses, contact with the eye is common, although not intended or desirable. In this case, the objective is a test that is a sensitive (as in the preceding paragraph), even if this results in a low incidence of false positives. Even a moderate irritant is not desired, but might be acceptable in certain cases (such as deodorants and depilatories), where the potential for eye contact is minimal.

Products that are not intended for personal care (such as soaps, detergents and drain cleaners) are approached from a different perspective. These products are not intended to be used in a manner that either causes them to get into eyes or makes that occurrence likely, but because a large population uses them and their modes of use do not include active measures to prevent eye contact (such as goggles or face shields), severe eye irritants must be identified accurately.

For agricultural chemicals, ocular exposure is never intended. However, unless rigorous steps are taken (which is almost never the case in the field), such exposure is unavoidable to a sizeable population. The desire here is to identify severe irritants or corrosives that require use of applicator systems or other methods of use that would preclude exposure. For ocular irritation, those chemicals used in food precessing are generally treated as industrial chemicals.

For industrial chemicals, eye irritation data are used primarily to fulfill labeling requirements for shipping and to provide hazard assessment information for accidental exposures and their treatment. The results of such tests do not directly affect the economic future of a material. It is desired to identify moderate and severe irritants accurately (particularly those with irreversible effects) and to determine if rinsing of the eyes after exposure will make the consequences of exposure better or worse. False negatives for mild reversible irritation are acceptable.

The needs and uses of these different communities in terms of ocular irritation data are summarized in Table 2. Historically, the philosophy underlying the test designs that were used to evaluate eye irritation made maximization of the biological response equivalent to being the most sensitive test. As this review of the objectives of the communities of interest has shown, the greatest sensitivity (especially at the expense of false positive findings, which is an unavoidable consequence) is not what is universally desired. As shall be seen later, maximizing the response in rabbits does not guarantee sensitive prediction of the results in humans.

As the matrix in Table 2 should make clear, for many of the users of such data, such a test system (although "blind" to mild and moderate irritants) would readily replace the need to use animal tests. At the same time, there are special cases where testing in the intact animal is the only means of detecting special case toxicities such as the exquisite lethality of parathion via the ocular route.

In summary, testing for eye irritation and other forms of ocular toxicity may be undertaken because of

- regulatory requirements
- liability concerns
- potential product selection
- need to plan plant construction and worker protection.

If, after a review of available data sources, these needs have not been met, then the question to be answered should be carefully defined in terms of intended product usage and potential human exposure. Then the necessary screen or test system can be selected to meet the defined need. The bulk of the remainder of this work is directed at selecting the appropriate test system.

STATE OF THE ART: *IN VIVO* TESTS

Over the 40 years since the publication of the Draize scoring system, it has become common practice to call all acute eye irritation tests performed in rabbits "the Draize eye test" (1944). However, since 1944, ocular irritation testing in rabbits has significantly changed. Clearly, there is no longer a single test design

TABLE 2
Matrix of Intended Product Use vs. Required Test Features for Ocular Irritation

	Features			
Types of Organization (Intended Product Use)	Desired Sensitivity (Lowest level of irritation that it is essential to detect)	Need to Evaluate Recovery and Effects of Timely Irrigation	Acceptable Incidence of False Positives	False Negatives
Pharmaceutical	Moderate	None	None	None
Cosmetic	Moderate	Recovery – High Irrigation – None	Minimal	None
Consumer Product[2] (Personal Use)	Moderate	Recovery – High Irrigation – Low	Minimal	None
Consumer Product (Household Use)	Severe	Medium to High	Low	Low to moderate None for sub-stantials
Agricultural Chemical	Severe	High	Low	None for severes
Industrial Chemical	Severe	High	Low	Low for sub-stantials None for severes

[2] Current FHSA regulations require that any consumer-used product (other than pharmaceuticals and cosmetics which are regulated by FDA), must be identified as to their potential to cause irritation as defined in this section.

that is used, and there are different objectives that are pursued by different groups using the same test. This lack of standardization has been recognized for some time and attempts have been made to address standardization of at least the methodological aspects of the test (such as how test materials are applied and scoring performed), if not the design aspects (such as numbers and sources of test animals). For the purpose of this text, we have therefore replaced the term "Draize test" with acute eye irritancy testing.

The common core design of the test has consisted of instilling either 0.1 ml of a liquid or 0.1 g of a powder (or other solid) onto one eye of each of six rabbits. The material is not washed out, and both eyes of each animal (the non-treated eye acting as a control) are graded according to the Draize scale (Table 3) at 24, 48 and 72 hours after test material instillation. The resulting scores are summed for each animal. The major subject of variations involve the use of three additional rabbits which have their eyes irrigated shortly after instillation of test material. There are, however, many variations of these two major design subsets (that is, with and without irrigation groups).

Even though the major objective of the Draize scale was to standardize scoring, it was recognized early that this was not happening, but that different people were "reading" the same response differently. To address this, two sets of standards (also called training guides, to provide guidance by comparison) have been published by regulatory agencies through the years. In 1965, the Food and Drug Administration (FDA, 1965) published an illustrated guide with color pictures as standards. In 1974, the Consumer Product Safety Commission (CPSC) published a second illustrated guide which provided 20 color photographic slides as standards. The Environmental Protection Agency (1979) also supported the development of a guide with color plates/slides, which is still available from NTIS (Falahee et al., 1981).

A second source of methodological variability has been in the procedure utilized to instill test materials into the eyes. There is a general consensus that the substance should be dropped into the cul-de-sac formed by gently pulling the lower eyelid away from the eye, then allowing the animal to blink and spread the material across entire corneal surface. In the past, however, there were other application procedures (such as placing the material directly onto the surface of the cornea).

There are also variations in the design of the "standard" test. Most laboratories observe animals until at least seven days after instillation and may extend the test to 21 days after instillation if any irritation persists (in fact, EPA labeling requires such an extension). These prolonged post-exposure observation periods are designed to allow for evaluation of the true severity of damage and for assessing the ability of the ocular damage to be repaired. The results of these tests are evaluated by a descriptive classification scale (Table 4) such as that described in NAS publication 1138 (NAS, 1977). This classification is based

TABLE 3
Scale of Weighted Scores for Grading
the Severity of Ocular Lesions [*] (Draize, 1944)

```
  I.  Cornea
      A.  Opacity-Degree of Density (area which is most dense is taken
            for reading)
            Scattered or diffuse area - details of iris clearly visible . . .   1
            Easily discernible translucent areas, details of iris slightly
              obscured  . . . . . . . . . . . . . . . . . . . . . . . . . . .    2
            Opalescent areas, no details of iris visible, size of pupil
              barely discernible  . . . . . . . . . . . . . . . . . . . . . .    3
            Opaque, iris visible  . . . . . . . . . . . . . . . . . . . . . .    4
      B.  Area of Cornea Involved
            One-quarter (or less) but not zero  . . . . . . . . . . . . . . .    1
            Greater than one-quarter, less than one-half  . . . . . . . . . .    2
            Greater than one-half, less than three-quarters . . . . . . . . .    3
            Greater than three-quarters up to whole area  . . . . . . . . . .    4
                    Scoring equals A x B x 5  Total maximum = 80

 II.  Iris
      A.  Values
            Folds above normal, congestion, swelling, circumcorneal ingestion
              (any one or all of these or combination of any thereof), iris
              still reacting to light (sluggish reaction is possible) . . . .    1
            No reaction to light, hemorrhage; gross destruction (any one or
              all of these) . . . . . . . . . . . . . . . . . . . . . . . . .    2
                    Scoring equals A x B   Total possile maximum = 10

III.  Conjunctivae
      A.  Redness (reers to palpegral conjuctival only)
            Vessels definitely injected above normal  . . . . . . . . . . . .    1
            More diffuse, deeper crimson red, individual vessels not easily
              discernible . . . . . . . . . . . . . . . . . . . . . . . . . .    2
            Diffuse beefy red . . . . . . . . . . . . . . . . . . . . . . . .    3
      B.  Chemosis
            Any swelling above normal (including nictitating membrane)  . . .    1
            Obvious swelling with partial eversion of the lids  . . . . . . .    2
            Swelling with lids about half closed  . . . . . . . . . . . . . .    3
            Swelling with lids about half closed to completely closed . . . .    4
      C.  Discharge
            Any amount different from normal (does not include small amount
              observed in inner canthus of normal animals)  . . . . . . . . .    1
            Discharge with moistening of the lids and hair just
              adjacent to the lids  . . . . . . . . . . . . . . . . . . . . .    2
            Discharge with moistening of the lids and considerable area
              around the eye  . . . . . . . . . . . . . . . . . . . . . . . .    3
                    Scoring (A + B + C) x 2   Total maximum = 20
```

```
The maximum total score is the sum of all scores obtained for the cornea,
iris and conjunctivae.

* Representative examples of various scores are presented in Figure 9A.
```

TABLE 4
Severity and Persistence (NAS, 1977)

INCONSEQUENTIAL OR COMPLETE LACK OF IRRITATION – Exposure of the eyes to a material under the specified conditions caused no significant ocular changes. No staining with fluorescein can be observed. Any changes that do occur clear within 24 hours and are no greater than those caused by normal saline under the same conditions.

MODERATE IRRITATION – Exposure of the eye to the material under the specified conditions causes minor, superficial, and transient changes of the cornea, iris, or conjunctivae as determined by external or slit–lamp examination with fluorescein staining. The appearance at the 24–hour or subsequent grading of any of the following changes is sufficient to characterize a response as moderate irritation: opacity of the cornea (other than a slight dulling of the normal luster), hyperemia of the iris, or swelling of the conjunctivae. Any changes that are seen clear within 7 days.

SUBSTANTIAL IRRITATION – Exposure of the eye to the material under the specified conditions causes significant injury to the eye, such as loss of the corneal epithelium, corneal opacity, iritis (other than a slight injection), conjunctivitis, pannus, or bullae. The effects clear within 21 days.

SEVERE IRRITATION OR CORROSION – Exposure of the eye to the material under the specified conditions results in the same types of injury as in the previous category and in significant necrosis or other injuries that adversely affect the visual process. Injuries persist for 21 days or more.

on the most severe response observed in a group of six nonirrigated eyes, and data from all observation periods are used for this evaluation. These will be examined more fully in the next section of this chapter.

Different regulatory agencies within the United States have prescribed slightly different procedures for different perceived regulatory needs (Gilman, 1982). These are looked at in more depth later in this chapter. There have also been a number of additional grading schemes, but these will not be reviewed here.

To fulfill the objectives of testing for different organizations, a number of basic text protocols have been developed and mandated by different regulatory groups. Table 5 gives an overview of these as previously presented by Gad and Chengelis (1988). Historically, the philosophy underlying these test designs made maximization of the biological response equivalent with having the most sensitive test. As our review of objectives has shown, the greatest sensitivity (especially at the expense of false positive findings, which is an unavoidable consequence) is not what is universally desired. As we shall see later, maximizing the response in rabbit does not *guarantee* sensitive prediction of the results in humans.

Methodological variations that are commonly used to improve the sensitivity and accuracy of describing damage in these tests are inspection of the eyes with a slit lamp and instillation of the eyes with a vital dye (or, most commonly, fluorescein) as an indicator of increase in permeability of the corneal barrier. These techniques and an alternative scoring system, which is more comprehensive than the Draize scale, are reviewed well by Ballantyne and Swanston (1977) and Chan and Hayes (1985).

Almost universally, the philosophy underlying these test designs equates maximization of the biological response with production of the most sensitive test. As our review of objectives has shown, the greatest sensitivity (especially at the expense of false positive findings, which is an unavoidable consequence) is not what is universally desired.

Ocular Irritation Test. The primary eye irritation test is intended to predict the potential for a single splash of chemical in the eye of a human to cause reversible and/or permanent damage. The basic study design for this test is shown diagrammatically in Figure 1. Since the introduction of the original Draize test 40 years ago, ocular irritation testing in rabbits has both developed and diverged. Indeed, clearly there is no longer a single test design that is used and there are different objectives that are pursued by different groups using the same test. This lack of standardization of at least the methodological aspects of the test, if not the design aspects.

TABLE 5
Regulatory Ocular Irritation Test Methods

Reference	Draize et al., 1944	FHSA*, 1964	NAS*, 1977	OECD*, 1981	IRLG*, 1981	CFR* 16, 1981 (CPSC*)	TOSCA*, 1982	FIFRA*, 1982**
Test Species	Albino rabbit	Same	Same[a]	Same	Same	Same	Same	Same
Age/Wt.	NS[b]	NS	Sexually mature/ less than 2 yrs. old	NS	Young adult/2.0	NS	NS	NS
Sex	NS	NS	Either	NS	Either	NS	NS	NS
Nos. of Animals/ Group	9	6–18	4 (min.)	3 (min.)	3 (prelim. test)[c]; 6	6–18	6	6
Test Agent Vol. and Method of instillation liquids	0.1 ml on the eye	Same as Draize	Liquids and solid; two or more diff. doses within the possible range of human exposure[d]	Same as Draize	Same as Draize	Same as Draize	Same as FHSA	Same as FHSA
Solids	NS	100 mg or 0.1 mL equivalent when this vol. weighs less than 100 mg; direct instillation into conjunctival sac	Mannner of applications should reflect probable route of accidental exposure	Same as FHSA	Same as FHSA	Same as FHSA	Same as FHSA	Same as FHSA
Aerosols[e]	NS	NS	Short burst at distance approximating self-induced eye exposure	1 sac burst sprayed at 10 cm	1 sac burst sprayed at approx. 4"	NS	As OECD	As OECD

Irrigation Schedule	At 2 sec (3 animals) and at 4 sec (3 animals follow-ing instilla-tion of test agent (3 animals remain non-irrigated)	Eyes may be washed after 24-hr. reading	May be con-ducted with separate experimental groups	Same as FHSA; in addition for substances found to be irritating; wash at 4 sec (3 animals) and at 30 sec (3 animals)	Same as FHSA	Same as FHSA	As FHSA	As FHSA
Irrigation Treatment	20 mL tap water (body temp.)	Sodium chloride solution (USP or equivalent)	NS	Wash with water for 5 min. using vol. and velocity of flow which will not cause injury	Tap water or sodium chloride solution (USP or equivalent	Same as FHSA	NS	NS
Examina-tion Times (post instilla-tion)	24 hr. 48 hr. 72 hr. 4 days 7 days	24 hr. 48 hr. 72 hr.	1 day 3 days 7 days 14 days 21 days	1 hr. 24 hr. 48 hr. 72 hr.	24 hr.[f] 48 hr. 72 hr.	24 hr. 48 hr. 72 hr.	As OECD	As OECD
Use of Fluor-escein	NS	May be applied after the 24 hr. reading (optional)	May be used	Same as FHSA	Same as FHSA	Same as FHSA	As FHSA	As FHSA

(Continued)

TABLE 5
Regulatory Ocular Irritation Test Methods

Reference	Draize et al., 1944	FHSA*, 1964	NAS*, 1977	OECD*, 1981	IRLG*, 1981	CFR* 16, 1981 (CPSC*)	TOSCA*, 1982	FIFRA*, 1982**
Use of Anesthetics	NS	NS	NS	May be used	May be sed	NS	May be used	May be used
Scoring and Evaluations	Draize et al., 1944	Modified Draize et al., 1944 or a slit lamp scoring system	CPSC, 1976	CPSC, 1976	CPSC, 1976	CPSC, 1976	(PSC, 1976)	PSC, 1976)

* FHSA = Federal Hazard Substances Act; NAS = National Academy of Sciences; OECD = Organization for Economic Cooperation and Development; IRLG = Interagency Regulatory Liaison Group; CFR = Code of Federal Regulations.

** Office Pesticide Assessment.

[a] Tests should be conducted on monkeys when confirmatory data are required.

[b] Not specified.

[c] If the substance produces corrosion, severe irritation or no irritation in a preliminary test with 3 animals, no further testing is necessary. If equivocal responses occur, testing on at least 3 additional animals should be performed.

[d] Suggested doses are 0.1 and 0.05 mL for liquids.

[e] Currently no testing guidelines exist for gases or vapors.

[f] Eyes may also be examined at 1 hr., 7, 14, and 21 days (at the option of the investigator).

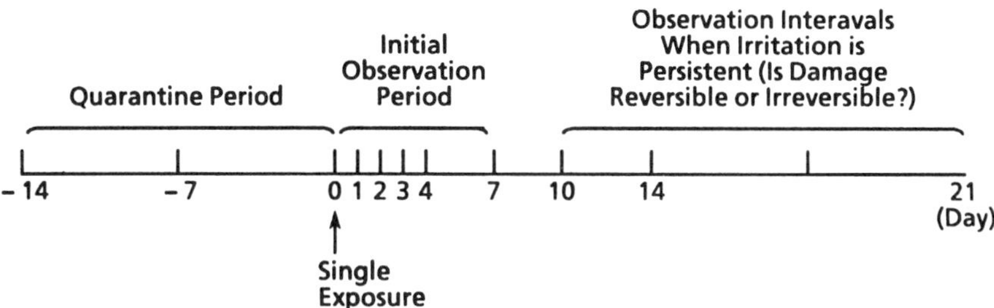

Figure 1.   Acute eye irritation study.

One widely used study design, which begins with a screening procedure as an attempt to avoid testing severe irritants or corrosives in animals, goes as follows:

A. *Test Article Screening Procedure* (presented diagrammatically in Figure 2).
  1. Each test substance will be screened in order to eliminate potentially corrosive or severely irritating materials from being studied for easy irritation in the rabbit.
  2. If possible, the pH of the test substance will be measured.
  3. A Primary Dermal Irritation (PDI) Study will be performed prior to the study.
  4. The test substance will not be studied for eye irritation, if the test substance is a strong acid (pH is 2.0 or less) or alkali (pH 11.0 or greater), and/or if the test substance is a severe dermal irritant (with a Primary Dermal Irritation Index - PDII - of 5 to 8) or causes corrosion of the skin.
  5. If it is predicted that the test substance does not have the potential to be severely irritating or corrosive to the eye, continue to Section B, Rabbit Screening Procedure.
B. *Rabbit Screening Procedure*
  1. A group of at least 12 New Zealand White rabbits of either sex are screened for the study. The animals are removed from their cages and placed in rabbit restraints. Care should be taken not to accidentally cause mechanical damage to the eye during this procedure.
  2. All rabbits selected for the study must be in good health; any rabbit exhibiting snuffles, hair loss, loose stools or apparent weight loss is rejected and replaced.
  3. One hour prior to instillation of the test substance, both eyes of each rabbit are examined for signs of irritation and corneal defects with a hand-held slit lamp. All eyes are stained with 2.0% sodium fluorescein

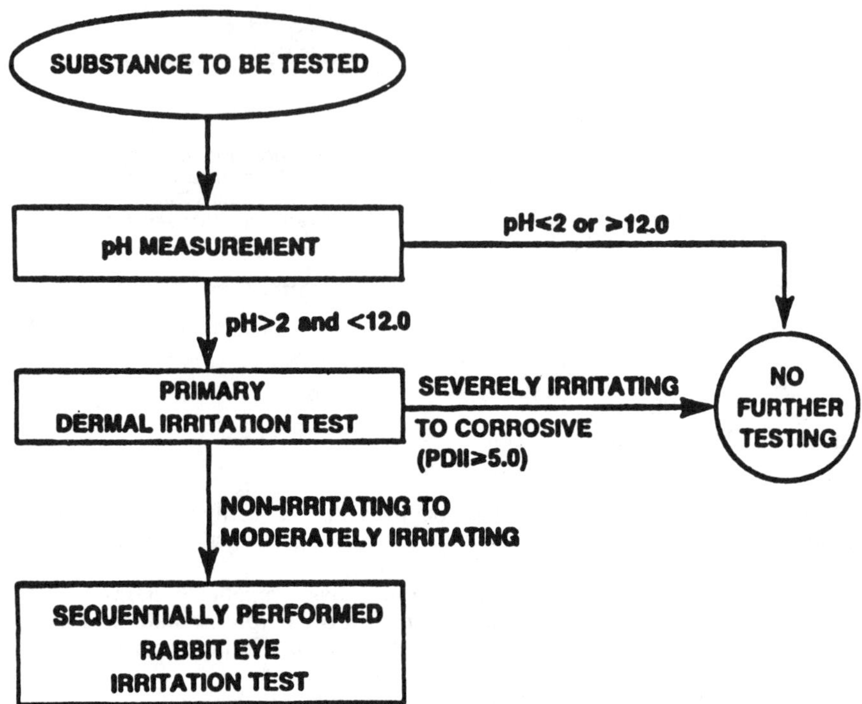

Figure 2.   Tier approach for eye irritation testing.

and examined to confirm the absence of corneal lesions.

Fluorescein Staining: Cup the lower lid of the eye to be tested and instill one drop of a 2% (in water) sodium fluorescein solution onto the surface of the cornea. After 15 seconds, the eye is thoroughly rinsed with physio-logical saline. The eye is examined, employing a hand-held long-wave ultraviolet illuminator in a darkened room. Corneal lesions, if present, appear as bright yellowish-green fluorescent areas.

4. Only 9 of the 12 animals are selected for the study. The 9 rabbits must not show any signs of eye irritation and must show either a negative or minimum fluorescein reaction (due to normal epithelial desquamation).

C. *Study Procedure*

1. At least one hour after fluorescein staining, the test substance is placed on one eye of each animal by gently pulling the lower lid away from the eyeball to form a cup (conjunctival cul-de-sac) into which the test material is dropped. The upper and lower lids are then gently held together for one second to prevent immediate loss of material.

2. The other eye remains untreated and serves as a control.

3. For testing liquids, 0.1 mL of the test substance is used. Note that this is the amount for the "standard test", which is believed to be excessive by the author.
4. For solids or pastes, 100 mg of the test substance is used.
5. When the test substance is in flake, granular, powder, or other particulate form, the amount that has a volume of 0.1 mL (after gently compacting the particles by tapping the measuring container in a way that will not alter their individual form) is used whenever this volume weighs less than 100 mg.
6. For aerosol products, the eye should be held open and the substance administered in a single, short burst for about one second at a distance of 4 inches directly in front of the eye. The velocity of the ejected material should not traumatize the eye. The dose should be approximated by weighing the aerosol can before and after each treatment. For other liquids propelled under pressure, such as substances delivered by pump sprays, an aliquot of 0.1 mL should be collected and instilled in the eye as for liquids.
7. The treated eyes of six rabbits are not washed following instillation of the test substance.
8. The treated eyes of the remaining three rabbits are irrigated for one minute with room temperature tap water, starting 20 seconds after instillation.
9. In order to prevent self-inflicted trauma by the animals immediately after instillation of the test substance, the animals are not immediately returned to their cages. After the test and control eyes are examined and graded at 1hr post-exposure, the animals are returned carefully to their respective cages.

D. *Observations*
   1. The eyes are observed for any immediate signs of discomfort after instilling the test substance. Blepharospasm and/or excessive tearing are indicate of irritating sensations caused by the test substance and the duration should be noted. Blepharospasm does not necessarily indicate that the eye will show signs of ocular irritation.
   2. Grading and scoring of ocular irritation are performed in accordance with Table 3. The eyes are examined and grades of ocular reactions are recorded.
   3. If signs of irritation persist at 7 days, readings are continued on days 10 and 14 after exposure or until all signs of reversible toxicity are resolved.
   4. In addition to the required observations of the cornea, iris and conjunctiva, serious effects (such as pannus, rupture of the globe or blistering of the conjunctivae) indicative of a corrosive action are reported.

5. Whether or not toxic effects are reversible depends on the nature, extent and intensity of damage. Most lesions, if reversible, will heal or clear within 21 days. Therefore, if ocular irritation is present at the 14-day reading, a 21-day reading is required to determine whether the ocular damage is reversible or non-reversible.

E. *Evaluation of Results*

The results can be evaluated by the following two methods:

1. Federal Hazardous Substances Act (FHSA) Regulations: (FHSA, 1964). Interpretation of data is made from the six test eyes which are not irrigated with water. Only data from days 1, 2 and 3 are used for this evaluation; data from the one-hour observation and days 4, 7 10, 14 and 21 are used. An animal shall be considered as exhibiting a positive reaction if the test substance products at any of the readings ulceration of the cornea (other than a fine stippling) [grade 1], or opacity of the cornea (other than a slight dulling of the normal luster) [grade 1], or inflammation of the iris (other than a slight deepening of the rugae or a slight circumcorneal injection of the blood vessels) [grade 1], or if such substance produces if the conjunctivae (excluding the cornea and iris), an obvious swelling with partial eversion of the lids [grade 2] or a diffuse crimson-red color with individual vessels not easily discernible [grade 2].

   The test shall be considered positive if four or more of the animals in the test group exhibit a positive reaction.

   If no or only one animal exhibits a positive reaction, the test is considered negative.

   If two or three animals exhibit a positive reaction, the test is repeated using a different group of six animals. The second test shall be considered positive if three or more of the animals exhibit a positive reaction.

   If only one or two of the animals in the second test exhibit a positive reaction, the test shall be repeated with a different group of six animals. Should a third test be needed, the substance will be regarded as an irritant if any animal exhibits a positive response. This FHSA scheme should be abandoned.

2. A modified Classification Scale of Ocular Responses is based on severity and persistence (derived from Green et al.). The most severe response seen in a group of six text animals is used for the classification. This scheme is presented in Table 4.

EXTENT OF *IN VIVO* TESTING

In order to generate a good approximation of how many rabbit eye irritation tests are performed in the U.S. and how many rabbits are used in the effort, a survey was designed and conducted specifically for an earlier review (Frazier et al., 1987). One hundred and ninety laboratories were identified as performing such tests in the U.S. and upon examination were classified into three categories which each included approximately a third of the total. These categories (called sectors) were contract research labs (58 facilities), pharmaceutical and cosmetic company labs (72 facilities), and chemical company labs (60 facilities, which include the labs of consumer product companies).

A random sample of ten facilities was then drawn by lot from each of the three sectors. These 30 organizations (representing, it should be noted, 16% of the total population) were then asked to provide information as to how many rabbit eye irritation tests they had performed in the last year, how many rabbits they had used in doing these tests, and what design modifications they might be employing. Specifically excluded were eye tests that were not intended to evaluate irritation. The results of this survey are presented in Table 6.

It should be noted that the "tests" performed annually in Table 6 include a variety of approaches, ranging from two-rabbit screens by many of the chemical company labs to a few 48-animal tests (for ophthalmologic agents) by pharmaceutical concerns. Two- and three-animal tests are screens means to detect severe irritants (or corrosives) only. This is why they are primarily used by the industrial chemical sector (such screens obviously address their objectives) or in fulfilling requirements of the OECD guidelines. Reduced numbers of animals are believed to not be suitable for a test designed to accurately do more than identify extreme and intermediate agents, as this would impair the predictive power of such tests due to the high degree of variability between animals (Bayard and Hehir, 1976). It should also be noted that this estimate of the total number of rabbits used in eye irritation testing is approximately one quarter of the Office of Technology Assessment's (OTA) estimate of the total number of rabbits used in all biomedical testing. The OTA estimate also includes animals used for dermal irritation and toxicity testing, teratogenicity, reproductive, pyrogenicity and pregnancy testing and teaching. It was expected that eye irritation testing would not constitute the majority usage of rabbits.

Current *in vivo* rabbit eye irritation tests also have the perceived advantages of being relatively inexpensive and of requiring minimal time from highly trained personnel. Performing large numbers of tests also leads to a substantial economy of mass effect, with significant reductions in the costs of doing tests. Depending on exactly how the tests are performed and on the local cost of the labor involved, a single material can be evaluated (including compliance with Good Laboratory Practices and the issuing of a final report, which generally account for at least 25% of the effort involved) for a cost of from 400 to 600 dollars. The times involved range from 10 to 30 person hours per test, with all but a small portion of this effort usually coming from the most junior technical staff.

TABLE 6
Rabbit Eye Tests

A. Tests Performed (Annual)

Sector	Range	Mean (X)	Weighing Factor (W)	Mean for Sector (X W)
Contract	10–800	258	(58)	14,964
Pharmaceutical	0–344	65	(72)	4,680
Chemical	28–155	83	(60)	4,980
		Estimated Total	(E)	24,624

B. Animals Used (Annual)

Sector	Range	Mean (X)	Weighing Factor (W)	Mean for Sector (X W)
Contract	90–4800	1520	(58)	88,160
Pharmaceutical	0–1032	234	(72)	16,848
Chemical	216– 488	296	(60)	17,760
			Total	122,768

W = No. of laboratory in sector is the weighing factor.

Notes to Table 4: Many of the laboratories surveyed reported using alternative techniques or test designs to reduce animal usage and discomfort. Some of these, in brief, are presented below.

A. Though one laboratory reported using 48 rabbits in a single eye irritation test, and a number of labs use a 9-animal design (6 non-washed and 3 washed), fully one-third of the laboratories use a screen or a sequential test design which reduces the number of animals per test in many (or even most) cases to 2-4 animals. One lab used both eyes, taking each as an independent variable and thus cutting in half the number of animals per test.

B. 10% of the labs have gone to a 0.01 ml test volume. Others are currently evaluating this change.

C. Five labs use the same animals for concurrent dermal and ocular irritation evaluations. Only one lab used the same animals for more than one eye irritation test; that lab performed a small number of tests.

D. Fully one-third of the laboratories perform some form of prescreen before performing an eye irritation study. Prescreens will be discussed later in this section.

E. Cost per test ranges from $325 to $1,500 each, depending on the details of the test performed and upon the nature of the personnel employed in performing tests.

In passing, it should also be pointed out that there is a degree of duplication in the testing that is performed - some materials are evaluated by more than one organization. This arises because eye testing data (indeed, all acute testing data) are not generally published. This lack of publication of acute results is due to two causes. First and foremost, the journals in toxicology do not generally believe that such data are of sufficient value to merit publication. The exception is the "battery" publication which presents a large number of results from such tests at one time, usually as support for a point of test interpretation or for changing test designs. The second reason such results are not published is due to concern of the proprietary nature of the materials tested. This concern has abated in recent years and, in fact, should continue to decline.

Adequacy of Current In Vivo Methods. To assess the adequacy of the currently employed eye irritation tests to fulfill the objectives behind their use, we must evaluate them in terms of (1) their accuracy (how well do they predict the hazard to humans); (2) can comparable results be obtained by different technicians and laboratories; and (3) reproducibility and precision within any single laboratory (how well a single lab can repeat tests and accurately evaluate standard or "control" materials). We should also consider what methods and designs have been developed and are being employed as modifications to rabbit eye irritation tests to improve their performance against these criteria.

Assessing the accuracy of rabbit eye irritation tests - or indeed, of any predictive test of eye irritation - requires that the results of such tests can be compared to what happens in man. Unfortunately, the human database available in the literature or resulting from controlled tests is not large. The concerns, however, have been present almost as long as the tests have been performed (McLaughlin, 1946).

There are substantial differences between the eyes of humans and those of rabbit - and indeed, of other species that have also been considered as test models. Beckley (1965) presented the following comparison of corneal thickness and area (as a percentage of the total area of the globe) of 4 species, as shown in Table 7.

The rabbit also has a different pH for its aqueous humor (7.6 vs. 7.1-7.3 for humans), a less effective tearing mechanism, and a nictitating membrane. Calabrese (1984) presents a comprehensive review of the anatomical and biochemical differences between the ocular systems of humans and rabbits.

Some have claimed that the rabbit, in the test as it is currently performed, is more sensitive than man. Many anionic formulations, for example, are severe rabbit eye irritants, but are nonirritants in humans. For other anionics, however, there is moderate human ocular irritation (such as with sodium dodecyl sulfate). However, the relative sensitivities vary from class to class of chemical.

TABLE 7
Corneal Thickness and Area

Species	Thickness (mm)	Area (%)
Man	0.53–0.54	7
Rabbit	0.4	25
Mouse	0.1	50
Rat	?	50

Alexander (1965) and Calabrese (1984) both have provided reviews of materials for which rabbits are more sensitive than man. McDonald et al. (1983) published a review of materials that were both more or less irritant in rabbits than in humans.

In the experience of the author (SCG), reviewing over a thousand materials, the prediction of irritancy in humans (as evaluated in medical and poison control center incidence reports) by rabbit eye tests (performed internally) is correct about 85% of the time. Approximately 10% of the time, the rabbit test tends to overpredict irritancy, while it underpredicts it less than 5% of the time. Swanston (1985) has also published a comparative review of 7 different species, including humans.

It should be noted, however, that rabbit eye tests do not detect ocular toxicities associated with some ocular anesthetics and eye drops (Andermann and Erhart, 1983).

The second concern, which has also been around as long as the test, is its reproducibility between laboratories. Weil and Scala published the most frequently cited study of intra-laboratory reproducibility of eye and skin irritation tests. Twenty-five labs evaluated a battery of 12 materials by a common protocol. The results showed variability between laboratories with a number of individual labs reporting consistently either more or less severe results than the other labs. A second comparative study, reported on by Marzulli and Rugles had ten laboratories test 7 liquid materials, 2 at a time, along with a control material. The materials were selected to be intermediate range eye irritants (5 materials) or nonirritants (2 materials). The labs utilized a common set of evaluation criteria, and were found to be quite consistent in properly classifying materials as irritants of nonirritants - a somewhat less stringent comparison of reproducibility than that employed by Weil and Scala. The causes and cures for such variability from lab to lab are multiple, but we have already mentioned differences in methodologies and evaluator training (to name just two major sources).

Since the Weil and Scala study, a number of authors, in addition to Marzulli and Rugles, have published comparative studies which have shown a greater degree of reproducibility, though they have not involved as large or diverse a population of evaluators. Some of these are summarized in Table 8 below.

Behind some of these differences in evaluating the reproducibility of the rabbit eye irritation test is a fundamental disagreement as to what such tests should do (or, more precisely, what kind of data they should generate). Many believe that the tests should serve to classify materials (into two or more categories, such as nonirritant/mild irritants/moderate irritants ...), while others believe it to be critical that a test effectively rank materials.

TABLE 8
Summary of Comparative Rabbit Eye Studies

	STUDY	RESULTS	REFERENCE
1.	3 Materials by 3 readers under 2 separate conditions	90% reproducibility of irritation/nonirritant classification	Bayard and Hehir (1976)
2.	7 materials evaluated in duplicate	Tests results reproducible	Williams et al. (1982)
3.	56 materials evaluated in 3 separate protocols	Each protocol reproducible - variations between tests by different protocols	Guillot et al. (1982)
4.	29 materials (detergents) evaluated in 2 rabbits, 1 monkey and 1 human test	Results for all non-human models were more severe than man, but low-volume rabbit test data were ranked comparable to human data	Freeberg et al. (1984)

Several authors have made the point that nonirritants and strong irritants are reproducibly predicted the best. For other materials, several authors have made the point that the use of concurrent reference materials (Gloxhuber, 1985) or twice annual refresher training of personnel doing scoring of results vs. a set of standards (McDonald et al., 1983) improves reproducibility of results and gives a set of standard results against which we can evaluate a drift in test or scoring practices.

Dunn et al. (1987) have presented data supporting the usefulness of early ocular examination in the design of rabbit eye irritation protocols by citing the incidence of transitory hyperemia of the iris associated with topical corneal and conjunctival exposure to 10 different substances. The iridial effects, as well as signs of conjunctival irritation and transitory corneal opacity, were detected by inclusion of a 1-hr. ocular examination. Five of the of 10 substances produced moderate eye irritation and the others produced inconsequential eye irritation when a description scale of ocular responses, based on severity, persistence and reversibility was applied. All would have been nonirritants by FHSA standards.

Limitations of the Rabbit Eye Test. The rabbit eye irritation test is designed to provide a range of information. First, what kinds of effects are to be expected and how severe are they? The Draize scale was never intended to provide a score such that the data are continuous and linear. That is, Draize scores are not such that a material with a score of 109 is distinguishably different than one with a score of 106. Rather, the results of scoring any one animal were intended to allow one to classify an agent as to its ability to cause or not cause irritation in that one animal.

Second, the test provides information as to rate of occurrence (or incidence) of irritation in animals. As demonstrated earlier, it is actually this information that is used to classify a material as an irritant or not.

Third, what is the time course or response, and are any/all adverse effects reversible? Earlier, the criteria for severity and reversibility were presented. Note that if a test is performed so that results (assuming there is irritation) are followed only for 72 hours as per the FHSA guidelines, the only classification of material that is possible is either irritant or nonirritant.

If one desires to more fully characterize and classify a material in this test system (such as a severe irritant), then one must either continue observations until the responses disappear or to 21 days (at which time most lesions can be determined to be either reversible or non-reversible). In certain cases (if the responses are extreme and test animals are in continued discomfort), a judgment can be made that effects will persist to 21 days, and the animals may be humanely terminated.

Fourth, for many uses, one may wish to know if there is a sensory warning response if a chemical is splashed into the eye. For some materials, such as dimethyl sulfoxide, methyl bromide and bis (2-chloroethyl) sulfate, no stinging or discomfort is caused - just damage to the eye later (Ballatyne and Swanston, 1977).

Finally, will washing or irrigation of the eye (the most common first aid procedure after an accidental exposure) alleviate the effects or make them worse?

There are modifications which have been proposed and adapted for the performance of rabbit eye irritation tests themselves that should be reviewed. These modifications have been directed at the twin objectives of making the tests more accurate in predicting human responses and at reducing both the use of animals and the degree of discomfort or suffering experienced by those that are used. Some of these modifications have already been discussed (under prescreening).

1. *Alternative Species:* Dogs, monkeys and mice (Swanston, 1985) have all been suggested as alternatives to rabbits that would be more representative of humans. Each of these, however, also has shown differences in responses compared to those seen in humans and pose additional problems in terms of cost, handling, lack of database, etc.

2. *Use of Anesthetics:* Over the years, a number of authors have proposed that topical anesthetics be administered to the eyes of rabbits prior to their use in the test. Both OECD and IRLG regulations allow such usage and the CPSC (1981) advocates their use. Numerous published (such as Falahee et al. 1981) and unpublished studies have shown that such use of anesthetics can interfere with test results (usually by increasing the severity and/or duration of eye irritation findings). However, the available literature remains mixed as to the scientific validity and/or advantages of using anesthetics in these tests.

3. *Decreased Volume of Test Material:* An alternative which has been proposed (and which our survey showed has been adopted by a number of laboratories) is using a reduced volume/weight of test materials.
   In 1980, Griffith et al. reported on a study in which they evaluated 21 different chemicals at volumes of 0.1, 0.03, 0.01 and 0.003 ml. These 21 chemicals were materials on which there were already human data. The volume reduction was found to not change the rank order of responses, and it was found that 0.01 ml (10 microliters) gave results which best mirrored those seen in man. In 1982, Williams et al. reported a comparison of 7 materials evaluated at 0.1 and 0.01 and found that the rank of results was not changed with the volume reduction while the responses were moderated.
   In 1984, Freeberg et al. published a study of 29 detergents (for which there were human data), each evaluated at both 0.1 and 0.01 ml test volumes in rabbits. The results of the 0.01 ml tests were reported to be more reflective of results in man. In 1986, Freeberg et al. published a further evaluation of

low vs. classical volume tests, in both humans and rabbits, and found that recovery times from low volume rabbit tests gave a better correlation with results seen in humans than classical volumes. In 1985, Walker reported on an evaluation of the low volume (0.01 ml) test, which assessed its results for correlation with those in humans based on the number of days until clearing of injury, and reported that 0.01 ml gave a better correlation than did 0.1 ml. There are only two objections to the low volume test. These are that we would lose a screen for exquisitely toxic materials (single drops of which in the eye will kill an animal, such as was reported for an organophosphonium salt by Dunn et al., 1982) and that there may be some classes of chemicals for which low volume tests may give less representative results.

The American Society of Testing and Materials (ASTM) has published the low volume method (Method E 1055-85) as a consensus standard procedure. It seems clear that this approach should be seriously considered by those performing *in vivo* eye irritation tests.

4. *Use of Prescreens:* This modification (presented in brief earlier) may also be considered a tier approach. Its objective is to avoid testing severely irritating or corrosive materials in many (or, in some case, any) rabbits. This approach entails a number of steps which should be considered independently.

First is a screen based on physicochemical properties. This usually means pH, but also should be extended to materials with high oxidation or reduction potentials (hexavalent chromium salts, for example).

Though the correlation between pH values (acids) and eye damage in the rabbit has not been found to be excellent, all alkalis (pH 11.5 or above) tested have been reported to produce opacities and ocular damage (Murphy et al., 1982). The lack of correlation of eye damage and low pHs is not limited to the rabbit, but, rather, is an inherent property of the more complex chemical reactivities of acids. Many laboratories now use pH cut-offs for testing of 2.0 or lower and 11.5 and 12.0 and higher. If a material falls under the provisions of these cut-offs (or is so identified due to other physicochemical parameters), then it should be (a) not tested in the rabbit eye and assumed to be corrosive; (b) evaluated in a secondary screen such as an *in vitro* cytotoxicity test or primary dermal irritation test (Jackson and Rutly, 1985); or (c) evaluated in a single rabbit before a full scale eye irritation test is performed. It should be kept in mind that the correlation of all the physicochemical screen parameters with acute eye test results is very concentration dependent, being good at high concentrations and marginal at lower concentrations (where various buffering systems present in the eye are meaningful).

The second commonly used type or level of prescreen is the use of primary dermal irritation (PDI) test results. In this approach, the PDI study is performed before the eye irritation study, and if the score from that study (called the primary dermal irritation index or PDII and ranging from 0 to 8) is above a certain level (usually 5.0 or greater), the same options already outlined for physicochemical parameter can be exercised. There is no universal agreement on the value of this prescreen. Gilman et al. (1983) did not find the PDII to be a good predictor, but made this judgment based on a relatively small data set and a cut-off PDII of 3.0 or above. In 1984 and 1985, Williams reported that severe PDII scores (5.0 or greater) predicted severe eye irritation responses in 39 of 60 cases. He attributed the false positives to possible over-prediction of potential human response by current PDI test procedures. On the other side, Gillot et al. reported good prediction of eye irritation based on PDIIs of 72 test materials.

5. *Staggered Study Starts:* Another approach, which is a form of screen, calls for starting the eye test in one or two animals, then delaying the dosing of the additional animals in the test group for 4 hours to a day. During this offset period, if a severe result is seen in the first one or two animals, the remainder of the test may be cancelled. This staggered start allows one to both limit testing severe eye irritants to a few animals and yet have confidence that a moderate irritant would be detected.
An integrated summary of the approach presented in these design modifications is shown in Figure 2.

6. *Use of Reduced Numbers of Animals:* Talsmer et al. (1988) have reported on a study of the adequacy of reducing the number of rabbits used per test. Data generated from 6-rabbit eye irritation tests of 155 various materials were used to determine the ability of irritation scores from all possible combinations of 5-, 4-, 3-, or 2-rabbit subsets to predict the Draize score derived from six rabbits. There are 930, 2325, 3100, and 2325 possible combinations of 155 studies for the 5-, 4-, 3-, and 2-rabbit subsets respectively. These classified materials using a four-level adjectival rating system based on (among other factors) the Draize score. Comparisons indicated that 5-, 4-, 3-, and 2-rabbit scores were in 98, 96, 94, and 91% agreement, respectively, with the classification assigned on the basis of the 6-rabbit score. The correlation coefficients for randomly selected subsets of 5-, 4-, 3-, and 2-rabbit scores versus the Draize score for six rabbits were 0.998, 0.996, 0.992, and 0.984, respectively. This study confirmed the findings of an earlier report by De Sousa et al., and indicates that a high level of accuracy can be obtained with reduced numbers of rabbits per test, particularly for more severe responses.

STATE OF THE ART: *IN VITRO* TESTS

The area of ocular irritancy has been the most active and fertile grounds for the development of true (*in vitro*) alternative tests since the beginning of the 1980's, Indeed, many of the *in vitro* tests now being evaluated for other endpoints (such as skin irritation and lethality) are adaptations of test systems first developed for eye irritation uses. A detailed review of each test system in this effort is beyond the scope of this volume. Frazier et al. (1987) performed such a review.

However, a working knowledge of the scope and basic assumptions behind such tests are essential. First, though, we must consider on a more formal basis why such tests are desirable.

Given the modifications that are being made to the traditional rabbit eye test, what are the advantages and disadvantages of the current rabbit eye tests in providing this information? The rationale for such tests and for seeking alternatives is presented in Table 9 and 10. These are modifications of lists originally published by Jackson (1983).

There are six major categories of approaches to *in vitro* eye irritation tests. The first five of these aim at assessing portions of the irritation response (alterations in tissue morphology, toxicity to individual component cell or tissue physiology, inflammation or immune modulation, and alterations in repair and/or recovery processes). These methods have the limitation that they assume that one of these component parts can or will predict effects in the complete organ system. A more likely case is that, while each may serve well to predict the effects of a set of chemical structures which have that component as a determining part of the ocular irritation response, a valid assessment across a broad range of structures will require the use of a collection or battery of such tests.

The sixth category contains tests which have little or no empirical basis, such as computer-assisted structure activity relationship models. These approaches can only be assessed in terms of how well (or poorly) they perform.   Table 11 presents an overview of all six categories and some of the component tests within them, updated from the assessment by Frazier et al., along with a single reference for each test.

Given that there are now some 60+ potential *in vitro* alternatives, the key points along the route to our eventual objective are thus: (1) how do we select the best candidates from this pool; (2) how do we want to use the resulting system (as a screen or test); and (3) how do we select, develop and validate the system (or systems) which will actually be used?

Before any of these steps, it is first necessary to decide criteria for what would constitute an ideal (or acceptable) test system.

Any useful test system must be sufficiently sensitive so that the incidence of false negatives is low. Clearly, a high incidence of false negatives is intolerable. In such a situation, large numbers of irritating or corrosive chemical agents would be carried through extensive additional testing, only to find that they possess undesirable toxicological properties after the expenditure of significant time and money. On the other hand, a test system which is overly sensitive will give rise to a high incidence of false positives, which will have the deleterious consequence of rejecting potentially beneficial chemicals. The "ideal" test will

TABLE 9
Rationale for Using Rabbit *(In Vitro)* Irritancy Tests

1. Provides whole animal and organ *in vivo* evaluation. The rabbit test assesses the inflammatory response of a complex organ composed of different tissues made up of numerous cell types. And when a tissue of an organ becomes inflamed, the whole animal responds.

2. Either neat chemicals or whole products (complex mixtures) can be tested. This allows us to address the complex chemical mixtures resulting from such processes as synthesis, augmentation, quenching and synergism.

3. Either concentrated or diluted products can be tested.

4. Yields data on the recovery and healing processes. A critical factor for a manufacturer to know in order to defend against liability suits.

5. Required screening test with the Federal Hazardous Substances Act (unless data area already available), Toxic Substances Control Act, Federal Insecticides, Fungicides and Rodenticides Act (FIFRA), and Organization for Economic Cooperation and Development (OECD).

6. Quantitative and qualitative test with the Draize Ocular Scoring Scale.

7. Amenable to modifications (irrigation, low volume, anesthetics), which were discussed in previous chapter.

8. Extensive database and cross-reference capability.

9. The ease of handling of the rabbit.

10. The eye of the albino rabbit presents a large surface of exposed globe for observation, and the lack of pigmentation in the iris makes it easier to interpret iritis.

11. Test is conservative, providing for maximum protection by erring on the side of overprediction of irritancy in man. With vision being our single most important sense, a greater degree of protection of these small and vulnerable organs is essential.

12. Test also provides screen for those agents which have usual or extremely systemic toxicity via the ocular route (Dunn et al., 1982).

TABLE 10
Rationale for Seeking *In Vitro*
Alternatives for Eye Irritancy Tests

1. Avoid whole animal and organ in vivo evaluation.

2. If strict Draize Scale is used, the rabbit in vivo test assesses only three eye structures (conjunctiva, cornea, iris). The Draize Eye Irritancy Test tells us nothing about cataracts, pain, discomfort, or clouding of the lens, for example.

3. Assesses only inflammation and immediate structural alterations produced by irritants (not sensitizers, photoirritants or photoallergens). Note, however, that the test was intended to evaluate only acute irritation. The in vivo test also does not necessarily evaluate any pain or discomfort.

4. Technician training and monitoring are critical (particularly due to the subjective nature of evaluation). (As it also will be with some in vitro test methods.)

5. If our objective is either the total exclusion of irritants or the identification of truly severe irritants on an absolute basis (that is, without false positives or negatives), rabbit eye tests do not perfectly predict results in humans. Some (such as Reinhardt and Schlatter, 1985) have claimed that these tests are too sensitive for such uses. The issue of relative sensitivity will be examined later in this section.

6. Clearly, however, there are structural and biochemical differences between rabbit and human eyes, which make extrapolation from one to the other difficult. For example, Bowman's membrane is present and well developed in man (8–12 mm thick) but not in the rabbit, possibly giving the cornea greater protection.

7. Lack of standardization.

8. Variable correlation with human results.

9. Large biological variability between experimental units.

10 Large, diverse and fragmented databases which are not readily comparable.

TABLE 11
Potential Alternatives for the Rabbit Eye Irritation Test

A. Morphology

    1. Enucleated Superfused Rabbit Eye System (Burton et al., 1981)

    2. Balb/c 3T3 Cells/Morphological Assays (HTD) (Borenfreund and Purner, 1984).

B. Cell Toxicity

    1. Adhesion/Cell Proliferation

        a. BHK Cell/Growth Inhibition (Reinhardt et al., 1985)

        b. BHK Cell/Colony Formation Efficiency (Reinhardt et al., 1985)

        c. BHK Cell/Cell Detachment (Reinhardt et al., 1985)

        d. SIRC Cell/Colony Forming Assay (North-Root et al., 1982)

        e. Balb/c 3T3 Cells/Total Protein (Shopsis and Eng, 1985)

        f. BCL-D1 Cells/Total Protein (Balls and Horner, 1985)

    2. Membrane Integrity

        a. LS Cells/Dual Dye Staining (Schaife, 1982)

        b. Thymocytes/Dual Fluorescent Dye Staining (Aeschbacher et al., 1986)

        c. LS Cells/Dual Dye Staining (Kemp et al., 1983)

        d. RCE-SIRC-P815-Yac-1/Cr Release (Shadduck et al., 1985)

        e. L292 Cells/Cell Viability/Hemolysis (Shadduck et al., 1987)

    3. Cell Metabolism

        a. Rabbit Corneal Cell Cultures/Plasminogen Activator (Chan, 1985)

        b. LS Cells/ATP Assay (Kemp et al., 1985)

        c. Balb/c 3T3 Cells/Uridine Uptake Inhibition Assay (Shopsis and Sathe, 1984)

        d. Balb/C 3T3 Cells/Neutral Red Uptake (Borenfreund and Purner, 1984)

        e. Hela Cells/Metabolic Inhibition Test (MIT-24) (Selling and Ekwall, 1985)

(Continued)

TABLE 11
Potential Alternatives for the Rabbit Eye Irritation Test

C. Cell and Tissue Physiology

   1. Epidermal Slice/Electrical Conductivity (Oliver and Pemberton, 1985)

   2. Rabbit Ileum/Contraction Inhibition (Muir et al., 1983)

   3. Bovine Cornea/Corneal Opacity (Muir, 1984)

   4. Proposed Mouse Eye/Permeability Test (Maurice and Singh, 1986)

D. Inflammation/Immunity

   1. Choriollantoic Membrane (CAM)

      a. CAM (Leighton et al., 1983)

      b. HET-CAM (Leupke, 1985)

      c. BECAM (Wetering and van Erp, 1987)

   2. Bovine Corneal Cup Model/Leukocyte Chemotatic Factors (Elgebaly et al., 1987)

   3. Rat Peritoneal Cells/Histamine Release (Jacaruso et al., 1985)

   4. Rat Peritoneal Mast Cells/Serotonin Release (Chasin et al., 1979)

   5. Rat Vaginal Explant/Prostaglandin Release (Dubin et al., 1985)

   6. Bovine Eye Cup/Histamine (Hm) and Leukotriene C4 (LT-C4) Release (Benassi et al., 1986)

E. Recovery/Repair

   1. Rabbit Corneal Epithelial Cells/Wound Healing (Jumblatt and Neufeld, 1985)

F. Other

   1. EYETEX Assay (Gordon and Bergmen, 1986)

   2. Computer Based/Structure Activity Relationship (SAR) (Enslein, 1984)

   3. Tetrahymena/Motility (Silverman, 1983)

fall somewhere between these two extremes and thus provide adequate protection without unnecessarily stifling development.

The "ideal" test should have an endpoint measurement which provides data such that dose-response relationships can be obtained. Furthermore, any criterion of effect must be sufficiently accurate in the sense that it can be used to reliably resolve the relative toxicity of two test chemicals which produce distinct (in terms of hazard to humans) yet similar responses. In general, it may not be sufficient to classify test chemicals into generic toxicity categories, such as "intermediate" toxicity, since a test chemical which falls in a given category, yet is borderline to the next more severe toxicity category, should be treated with more concern than a second test chemical which falls at the less toxic extreme of the same category. Therefore, it is useful for a test system to be able to rank test chemicals accurately within any general toxicity category.

The endpoint measurement of the "ideal" test system must be objective. This is important so that a given test chemical will give similar results when tested using the standard test protocol in different laboratories. If it is not possible to obtain reproducible results in a given laboratory over time or between various laboratories, then the historical database against which new test chemicals are evaluated will be time/laboratory dependent. Along these lines, it is important for the test protocol to incorporate internal standards to serve as quality controls. Thus, test data could be represented utilizing a reference scale based on the test system response to the internal controls. Such normalization, if properly documented, could reduce inter-test variability.

The test results for a given chemical should be reproducible both intrinsically (within the same laboratory over time) and extrinsically (between laboratories). If this condition is not satisfied, then there will be significant limitations on the application of the test system since it could potentially produce conflicting results. From a regulatory point of view, this possibility would be highly undesirable.

Alternatives to the *in vivo* eye tests basically should be designed to evaluate the acute toxic response of the ocular system following a single exposure to the test chemical. Although there are certain variations of the Draize eye test utilized to evaluate repeated exposures to a test agent, they are not the basis of the original test. However, for agents which may enter the conjunctival sac repeatedly, such as facial cosmetics, it would be desirable if the test protocol could be modified to accommodate such an exposure sequence. This would certainly be a useful property of a test protocol, but not an essential feature.

From a practical point of view, there are several additional features of the "ideal" test which should be satisfied. The test should be rapid so that the turnaround time for a given test chemical is reasonable. Obviously the speed of the test and the ability to conduct tests on several chemicals simultaneously will determine the overall productivity. The test should be inexpensive so that it is economically competitive with current testing practices. And finally, the technology should be easily transferred from one laboratory to another without excessive capital investment for test implementation. It should be kept in mind that although some of these practical considerations may appear to present formidable limitations for a given test system at the present time, the possibility of future developments in testing technology could overcome these obstacles.

This brief discussion of the characteristics of the "ideal" test system provides a framework for evaluation of alternative test systems in general. No test system is likely to be "ideal". Therefore, it will be necessary to weigh the strengths and weaknesses of each proposed test system in order to reach a conclusion on how "good" a particular test is. The next section will present the basis for the specific test evaluation.

Criteria for Test Evaluation. Many test systems described in the literature (Table 11) have been proposed as alternatives to eye irritancy testing. In order to compare these potential alternative tests, it is necessary to establish a set of yardsticks which can be used to evaluate each test system. Criteria which should be considered for such a selection process are described below.

The actual evaluation of individual test systems is divided into four categories: (I) test purpose, (II) logistics, (III) scientific and (IV) economic.

(I) Test Purpose: As described at the beginning of this discussion, any evaluation of a potential test method must start with a firm understanding of the objectives behind test conduct. Establish the needs of the "community of interest".

(II) Logistics: For a test system to be of practical use, it is essential that it meet criteria with respect to: its ability to be standardized; whether it is transferable between laboratories; and whether components of the system are available commercially. Although at first glance these three aspects appear to be independent they are in fact strongly interdependent. The greater the ability to standardize a test protocol the more easily it can be transferred between laboratories. If components of the test system are available commercially, it will be more easily standardized. Thus, one finds that generally there is a strong relationship between commercial availability of components of the test system and whether it meets the logistics criteria.

From this point of view, most test systems can be divided into two components: the biological component and the non-biological component. The biological component is the cell culture, tissue or organ which is used to evaluate the toxicity of the chemical agent. The non-biological component consists of everything else and can be subdivided into those elements which support the biological component and those elements which are involved in the endpoint evaluation. It should be noted that the non-biological components of a test system may include materials derived from biological systems, such as fetal calf serum or antibodies.

(III) Scientific: This portion of an evaluation looks at the scientific merit of the test system. The first question to be addressed is the nature of the test; i.e., does the endpoint measured evaluate a critical step in the inflammatory/irritation response (is it a mechanistic based test); or does it measure a parameter which merely correlates with the response (a correlation based test). This is an important point in terms of acceptance of the test by regulatory agencies since mechanistic tests should be more readily interpretable. Secondly, the endpoint of the test will be evaluated as to whether it is subjective or objective. If it is subjective then the grading scale will be evaluated. The second step in the scientific evaluation is to determine the performance of the test as measured by its correlation with the results of the *in vivo* eye test in either animals or man. This allows a comparison to be made with a relatively large database in the case of animal data and, where the data are available, the results for a given test can be correlated with the human experience. In general, these data should be compared on the basis of rank correlations. No attempt can generally be made to correlate these data on a quantitative basis.

(IV) Economics: This deals with factors which determine the cost of the test system. The major components of an analysis include the operational cost of the test per full evaluation of a specific test chemical, the time it takes to carry a test chemical completely through an evaluation and the capital investment for facilities required to perform the test. The operational costs include technician time for maintenance of the test system and the biological component, professional time for evaluation of results, costs for non-biological components and technician time for endpoint analysis. Qualitative estimates (high, low, mid) should also be considered with respect to cost since it is generally impractical to attempt quantitative estimates at this stage.

The time required to conduct a particular test consists of 3 components: (a) the time to prepare stock cultures of the biological component in a format suitable for performing the test, (b) the actual time involved in the test procedure, and (c) the time for endpoint analysis. For each system, the time commitment for each step in the process must be estimated. A rapid test is any one which can be completed within three days from the time the biological component is prepared and ready for test initiation to the completion of test data analysis.

Considerations in Adopting New Test Systems. Conducting toxicological investigations in three or more species of laboratory animals is generally accepted as being a prudent and responsible practice in developing a new chemical entity, especially one that is expected to receive widespread use and to have exposure potential over human lifetimes. Adding a second or a third species to the testing regimen offers an extra measure of confidence to the toxicologist and the other professionals who will be responsible for evaluating the associated risks, benefits and exposure limitations or protective measures. Although undoubtedly broadening and deepening a compound's profile of toxicity, the practice of enlarging on the number of test species is, as has been demonstrated in multiple points in the literature (Gad and Chengelis, 1988, for example), an indiscriminate scientific generalization. Moreover, such a tactic is certain to generate the problem of species specific toxicoses; that is, a toxic response or an inordinately low biological threshold for toxicity is evident in one species or strain, while all other species examined are either unresponsive or strikingly less sensitive. The investigator confronting such findings must be prepared to address the all important question, "Are humans likely to react positively or negatively to the test agent under similar circumstances?"

Assuming that numerical odds prevail and humans automatically fit into the predominant category, whether on the side of being safe or at risk, would be scientifically irresponsible. Far from being an irreconcilable nuisance, however, such a confounded situation can be an opportunity to advance more quickly into the heart of the search for predictive information. This is the case discussed in the earlier section on cross-species extrapolation. A species-specific toxicosis can frequently contribute toward better understanding of the general case if the underlying biological mechanism either causing or enhancing toxicity is defined and especially if it is discovered to uniquely reside in the sensitive species.

A mention of species-specific toxicosis usually implies that either different metabolic pathways for converting an excreting xenobiotic or anatomical differences are involved. The design of our current tests appears to serve society reasonably well (i.e., significantly more times than not) in identifying hazards that would be unacceptable. However, the process can just as clearly be improved from the standpoints of both improving our protection of society and doing necessary testing in a manner that uses fewer animals and uses these fewer animals in a more humane manner.

In Vitro Models. In vitro models, at least as screening tests, have been with us in toxicology for some twenty years now. The last five to ten years have brought a great upsurge in interest in such models. This increased interest is due to economic and animal welfare pressures and technological improvements.

Criteria against which an *in vitro* model should be evaluated for its suitability in replacing (partially or entirely) an accepted *in vivo* model are incorporated in the process detailed in Table 12.

In vitro systems *per se* have a number of limitations which can contribute to their not being acceptable models. Some of these reasons are detailed in Table 13.

TABLE 12
Multistage Scheme for the Development, Validation and
Transfer of *In Vitro* Test System Technology in Toxicology

STAGE I.   STATEMENT OF TEST OBJECTIVE

A.   IDENTIFY EXISTING TEST SYSTEM AND ITS STRENGTHS AND WEAKNESSES

B.   CLEARLY STATE OBJECTIVES FOR ALTERNATIVE TEST SYSTEM

C.   IDENTIFY POTENTIAL ALTERNATIVE TEST SYSTEM

STAGE II.   DEFINE DEVELOMENTAL TEST DESIGN

A.   IDENTIFY RELEVANT VARIABLES

B.   EVALUATE EFFECTS OF VARIABLES ON TEST SYSTEM

C.   REDESIGN TEST TO OPTIMIZE TEST PERFORMANCE

D.   UNDERSTAND WHAT THE TEST DOES IN A FUNCTIONAL SENSE

(1) Is it a simulation of an in vivo event?

(2) Is this simply a response to the presence of the agent?

(3) Is this a functional step or link in that event?

(4) Is this an event or a property mechanistically linked to that
event or some intermediate stage?

(5) Is this an effect on some structure or function analogous to the
in vivo structure or function?

STAGE III.   EVALUATE PERFORMANCE ON OPTIMUM TEST

A.   DEVELOP BATTERY OF KNOWN POSITIVE AND NEGATIVE RESPONSE MATERIALS OF
DIVERSE STRUCTURE

B.   USE OPTIMUM TEST DESIGN TO EVALUATE BATTERY OF "KNOWNS" UNDER "BLIND"
CONDITIONS

C.   COMPARE CORRELATION OF TEST RESULTS OF THOSE OF OTHER TEST SYSTEMS AND
TO REAL CASE OF INTEREST - RESULTS IN HUMANS

(Continued)

TABLE 12
Multistage Scheme for the Development, Validation and Transfer of *In Vitro* Test System Technology in Toxicology

---

STAGE IV.   TECHNOLOGY TRANSFER

A.   PRESENT AND PUBLISH RESULTS THROUGH PROFESSIONAL MEDIA (SOCIETY MEETINGS,
PEER-REVIEWED JOURNALS)

B.   PROVIDE HANDS-ON TRAINING TO PERSONNEL FROM OTHER FACILITIES AND
FACILITATE THEIR PERFORMING INTERNAL EVALUATIONS OF TEST METHODS

STAGE V.   VALIDATION

A.   ARRANGE FOR TEST OF CODED SAMPLES IN MULTIPLE LABS (I.E., INTERLABORATORY
VALIDATION)

B.   COMPARE, PRESENT AND PUBLISH RESULTS

STAGE VI.   CONTINUE TO REFIRNE AND EVLAUATE TEST SYSTEM PERFORMANCE
AND UTILIZATION

A.   CONTINUALLY STRIVE FOR AN UNDERSTANDING OF WHY THE TEST "WORKS" AND ITS
RELEVANCE TO EFFECTS IN MAN

B.   REMAIN SKEPTICAL.   WHY SHOULD ANY ONE OF US BE THE ONE TO MAKE THE BIG
BREAKTHROUGH?   CLEARLY THERE IS SOME BASIC FLAW IN THE DESIGN OR CONDUCT OF
THE STUDY WHICH HAS GIVEN RISE TO THESE PROMISING RESULTS.   DOUBT, CHECK
AND QUESTION; THEN LET YOUR MOST SEVERE CRITIC REVIEW THE DATA; THEN GO
TO A NATIONAL MEETING AND GIVE A PRESENTATION; THEN GO BACK HOME AND
DOUBT, CHECK AND QUESTION SOME MORE!

TABLE 13
Possible Interpretations when *In Vitro* Data Do Not Predict Results of *In Vivo* Studies

1. Chemical is not absorbed at all or is poorly absorbed in in vivo studies.

2. Chemical is well absorbed but is subject to first-pass effect in liver.

3. Chemical is distributed so that less (or more) reaches the receptors than would be predicted on the basis of its absorption.

4. Chemical is rapidly metabolized to an active or inactive metabolite that has a different profile of activity and/or different duration of action than the parent drug.

5. Chemical is rapidly eliminated (e.g., through secretory mechanisms).

6. Species of the two test systems used are different.

7. Experimental conditions of the in vitro and in vivo experiments differed and may have led to different effects than expected. These conditions include factors such as temperature or age, sex, and strain of animal.

8. Effects elicited in vitro and in vivo by the particular differ in their characteristics.

9. Tests used to measure responses will probably differ greatly for in vitro and in vivo studies, and the types of data obtained may not be comparable.

10. The in vitro study did not use adequate controls (e.g., pH, vehicle used, volume of test agent given, samples taken from sham-operated animals).

11. In vitro data cannot predict the volume of distribution in central or in peripheral compartments.

12. In vitro data cannot predict the rate constants for chemical movement between compartments.

13. In vitro data cannot predict the rate constants of chemical elimination.

14. In vitro data cannot predict whether linear or nonlinear kinetics will occur with specific dose of a chemical in vivo.

15. Pharmacokinetic parameters (e.g., bioavailability, peak plasma concentration, half-life) cannot be predicted based solely on in vitro studies.

16. In vivo effects of chemical are due to an alteration in the higher order integration of an intact animal system, which cannot be reflected in a less complex system.

At the same time there are substantial potential advantages in using *in vitro* systems. These advantages of using cell or tissue culture in toxicological testing are isolation of test cells or organ fragments from homeostatic and hormonal control, accurate dosing, and quantitation of results. It is important to devise a suitable model system which is related to the mode of toxicity of the compound. Tissue and cell culture have been used in two very different ways in screening studies. Firstly, it has been used to examine a particular aspect of the toxicity of a compound in relation to its toxicity *in vivo*. Secondly, it has been used as a form of rapid screening to compare the toxicity of a group of compounds.

NEAR TERM ADVANCES: A MIXED BATTERY

From the preceding sections several points should be clear.

1. Ocular irritation testing should not continue to be performed as it has been.
2. There are no generally accepted *in vitro* test systems immediately available to replace all (or, indeed, any) of the *in vivo* testing requirements.
3. There are some steps which can be taken to move development and acceptance of *in vitro* systems along.
4. There are some modifications to current in vivo testing methods which both can and should be adopted.

Before developing these points, however, one must consider the needs of the communities of interest responsible for testing and understand the concept of a screen (as opposed to a definitive test).

For the pharmaceutical industry (with the exception of the case of contact lenses, which will not be discussed here), eye irritation testing is done when the material is intended to be put into the eye as a means or route of application or for ocular therapy. There are a number of special tests applicable to pharmaceuticals or medical devices that are beyond the scope of this volume, as they are not intended to assess potential acute effects or irritation. In general, however, an eye irritation test that is used by this group must be both sensitive and accurate in predicting the potential to cause irritation in humans. Failing to identify human ocular irritants (lack of sensitivity) is to be avoided, but of equal concern is the occurrence of false positives.

The cosmetics and toiletries industry is similar to the pharmaceutical industry in that the materials of interest are frequently intended for repeated application in the area of the eye. In such uses, contact with the eye is common although not intended or desirable. In this case, the objective is a test that is a sensitive (as in the preceding paragraph), even if this results in a low incidence of false positives. Even a moderate irritant is not desired, but might be acceptable in certain cases (such as deodorants and depilatories) where the potential for eye contact is minimal.

Consumer products that are not intended for personal care (such as soaps, detergents and drain cleaners) are approached from a different perspective. These products are not intended to be used in a manner that either causes them to get into eyes or makes that occurrence likely, but because a large population uses them and their modes of use do not include active measures to prevent eye contact (such as goggles or face shields), severe eye irritants must be identified accurately.

For agricultural chemicals, ocular exposure is never intended. However, unless rigorous steps are taken (which is almost never the case in the field), such exposure is unavoidable to a sizeable population. The desire here is to identify severe irritants or corrosives that require use of applicator systems or other methods of use that would preclude exposure. For ocular irritation, those chemicals used in food processing are generally treated as are industrial chemicals.

For industrial chemicals, eye irritation data are used primarily to fulfill labeling requirements for shipping and to provide hazard assessment information for accidental exposures and its treatment. The results of such tests do not directly affect the economic future of a material. It is desired to identify moderate and severe irritants accurately (particularly those with irreversible effects) and to know if rinsing of the eyes after exposure will make the consequences of exposure better or worse. False negatives for mild reversible irritation are acceptable.

The needs and uses of these different communities in terms of ocular irritation data were summarized previously in Table 2. Historically, the philosophy underlying the test designs that were used to evaluate eye irritation made maximization of the biological response equivalent to being the most sensitive test. As this review of the objectives of the communities of interest has shown, the greatest sensitivity (especially at the expense of false positive findings, which is an unavoidable consequence) is not what is universally desired. As has been demonstrated, maximizing the response in rabbits does not guarantee sensitive prediction of the results in humans.

Concept of Screens. Screens are simple tests which try to answer single questions with great sensitivity (but not necessarily marked specificity). Many of the currently proposed *in vitro* systems show immediate promise as screens. As such, they would be employed to rapidly and efficiently identify those materials which were clearly strong irritants or corrosives, and therefore did not need further evaluation.

Until in vitro tests are further developed and accepted, then, what should be utilized is a mixed tier approach. The tier approach presented earlier in Figure 2 is one form which can be (and is being) utilized currently, but this can be improved on. For the near term, a better system could be used which employs a mixed series of screening steps. Such a system would have the following stages.

I. *In Vitro* Screen
   a. Extremely active compounds in a cytotoxicity assay should be considered strong irritants (or worse) and classified/handled as such. Note that this should also serve to identify (among others) the same compounds as the current pH screen, and therefore that step is not required.
   b. Less active or inactive compounds would pass on, unless the testing need was only to identify I(a) type compounds (in which case testing is complete).

II. Primary Dermal Irritation
   a. Severely irritating to corrosive compounds should be treated as I(a) above.
   b. Mild to nonirritants should be treated as I(b).

III. Staggered Eye Irritation Test
Using a low volume form test, materials would be evaluated using a single animal. If no irritation was seen at 24 hours, a second (and 24 hours later, a third) rabbit would be added to the test. Clear positive findings would stop the test.

FAR HORIZONS; AND HOW TO GET THERE

Clearly great progress has been made both in improving practices as to the conduct of eye irritation tests in intact rabbits and in developing an array of promising *in vitro* candidates for replacement of the *in vivo* test.

Where we would like to be is to have in place (that is, accepted and used by industry and regulatory agencies) one or a battery of *in vitro* systems which would reduce the need for intact animal testing to the rare case of opthalmic pharmaceuticals. And to have duplicate testing of materials reduced to a minimum. It does not appear that we are any closer to these being the case than we were in 1985, and no progress towards these specific objectives is immediately apparent. How does the science and practice of toxicology go about getting to this point?

The critical missing step is that there needs to be a collaborative interlaboratory validation of candidate *in vitro* alternative tests. In this effort, a select committee of individuals knowledgeable in the field would establish two "panels" of test compounds. Each panel would contain a representative variety of chemical structures (i.e., not limited to alcohols, surfactants, acids, etc.) with known irritant potential in humans and rabbits.

Some of these compounds would be corrosives, some strong irritants, some non-irritants, etc. Some of the materials would be mixtures. Each panel compound would be analyzed. The first panel would contain some 20 materials, the second some 30 more. A central repository would package, code, label, and disburse samples of each panel.

Those investigators who have candidate test systems would be invited to participate in the validation effort. All those that accepted would be provided with a randomly coded set of panel A compounds. Those who elect not to participate should be published/reported as having turned down the opportunity to participate. Once all the laboratories who elect to participate have returned data, (and completion and reporting of data should be required in a specified period - say three months) the data can be analyzed and test systems evaluated as "go" or "no go", based on such performance and the previously identified logistical and economic factors.

"Go" test systems would then be used to evaluate panel B compounds. This additional performance information should be sufficient to allow identification of the best (or equivalent) single test or battery of tests. The total effort should then be published with the recommendations of the committee as to use of the tests. This would then form the basis to cause both industry and government to use and accept the new testing schemes. A major step towards reducing duplicate testing would be providing a mechanism for publication of acute testing data. A reference journal dedicated to the purpose would seem to be a viable course, and this possibility is currently being explored.

REFERENCES

AESECHBACHER, M. REINHARDS, C.A. and ZBINDEN, G. (1986). A rapid cell membrane permeability test using fluorescent dyes and flow cytometry. Cell Biol. Toxicol.

ALEXANDER, P. (1965). Evaluation of the irritation potential of shampoos and conditioning rinses. Specialties 9:33-37

AMERICAN CONFERENCE OF GOVERNMENTAL INDUSTRIAL HYGIENISTS (ACGIH) (1986). Documentation of the Threshold Limit Values, Fifth Edition, Cincinnati, OH.

AMERICAN INDUSTRIAL HYGIENE ASSOCIATION (AIHA) (1980). Hygienic Guide Series. Volumes I and II, AIHA, Akron, OH.

ANDERMANN, G. and ERHART, M. (1983). Meth. and Find. Exptl. Clin. Pharmacol. **5**: 321-333.

BALLANTYNE, B. and SWANSTON, D.W. (1977). The scope and limitations of acute eye irritation tests. Current Approaches in Toxicology, (B. Ballantyne, ed.), pp. 139-157, John Wright & Sons, Bristol.

BALLS, M. and HORNER, S.A. (1985). The FRAME interlaboratory program on *in vitro* cytotoxicology. Fd. Chem. Toxic. **23**:205-213.

BARNHART, E.R. (1987). Physicians Desk Reference, Medical Economics Company, Oradell, NJ.

BYARD, S. and HEHIR, R.M. (1976). Evaluation of Proposed Changes in the Modified Draize Rabbit Irritation Test. Soc. Toxicol. 15th Meeting, Atlanta, GA. Abstract 225.

BECKLEY, J.H. (1965). Comparative Eye Testing: Man vs. Animal. Tox. App.Pharm. 7:93-101.

BENASSI, C.A., ANGI, M.R., SALVALAIO, L. and BETTERO, A. (1986). Histamine and leukotriene C4 release from isolated bovine scherachroid complex: A new *in vitro* ocular irritation test, Chimica Agg.

BORENFREUND, E. and PEURNER, J.A. (1984). A simple quantitative procedure using monolayer cultures for cytotoxicity assays (HTD/NR-NE). J. Tissue Culture Methods **9**:7-10.

BURTON, A.B.G., YORK, M. and LAWRENCE, R.S. (1981). The *in vitro* assessment of severe eye irritants. Fd. Cosmet. Toxicol. **19**:471-480.

CALABRESE, E.J. (1984). Principles of Animal Extrapolation, pp. 391-402. John Wiley & Sons, New York.

CHAN, K.Y. (1985). An *in vitro* alternative to the Draize test. In *In Vitro* Toxicology: Alternative Methods in Toxicology (A.M. Goldberg, ed.), Vol. 3, pp. 405-422. Mary Ann Liebert, Inc., New York.

CHAN, P.K. and HAYES, A.W. (1985). Assessment of chemically induced ocular toxicity: A survey of methods. In Toxicology of the Eye, Ear and Other Special Senses (A. W. Hayes, ed.), pp. 103-143. Raven Press, New York.

CHASIN, M., SCOTT, C., SHAW, C. and PERSICO, F. (1979). A new assay for the measurement of mediator release from rat peritoneal in most cells. Int. Archs. Allergy Appl. Immun. **58**:1-10.

CLAYTON, D.G. and CLAYTON, F.E. (1981). Patty's Industrial Hygiene and Toxicology, 3rd Ed., Volumes 2A, 2B, and 2C. John Wiley & Sons, New York.

CPSC (1974). Illustrated Guide for Grading Eye Irritation Caused by Hazardous Substances, 16 CFR 1500.

DE SOUSA, D.J., ROUSE, A.A. and SMOLON, W.J. (1984). Statistical consequences of reducing the number of rabbits utilized in eye irritation testing. Data on 67 petrochemicals. Toxicol. Appl. Pharmacol. **76**:234-242.

DRAIZE, J.H., WOODARD, G. and CALVERY, H.O. (1944). Methods for the study of irritation and toxicity of substances applied topically to the skin and mucous membranes. J. Pharmacol. Exp. Ther. **82**:377-390.

DUBIN, N.H. and DE BLASI, M.C., et al. (1984) Development of an *in vitro* test for cytotoxicity in vaginal tissues: Effect of ethanol on prostanoid release. In Acute Toxicity Testing: Alternative Approaches (A.M. Goldberg, ed.), Alternative Methods in Toxicology, Vol. 2, pp. 127-138. Mary Ann Liebert, Inc., New York.

DUNN, B.J., GAD, S.C., POWERS, W.J., WALSH, R.D. and NICHOLS, C.W. (1987). Importance of early ocular examination to detect transitory irritation. J. Toxicol.-Cut. & Ocular Toxicol. **6**:193-200.

DUNN, B.J. NICHOLS, C.W. and GAD, S.C. (1982). Acute dermal toxicity of two quarternary organophosphonium salts in the rabbit. Toxicology **24**:245-250.

ELGEBALY, S.A., FOROUHR, F. and KREUTZER, D.L. (1987). *In vitro* protection of cornea-derived leukocytic chemotactic factors as indicators of corneal inflammation. In *In Vitro* Toxicology: Approaches to Validation. (A.M. Goldberg, ed.), pp. 257-268. Mary Ann Liebert, Inc., New York.

ENSLEIN, K. (1984). Estimation of toxicology endpoints by structure-activity relationships. Pharmacol. Rev. **36**:131-134.

EPA (1979). Acute Toxicity Testing Criteria for New Chemical Substances. EPA 560/13-79-009, 9-14.

EPA (1986). Guidelines for Carcinogen Risk Assessment. Fed. Reg. **51**:185 (September 24), 33992-34054.

FALAHEE, K.J., ROSE, C.S., OLIN, S.S. and SEIFRIED, H.E. (1981). Eye Irritation Testing: An Assessment of Methods and Guideliens for Testing Materials for Eye Irritancy. Office of Pesticides and Toxic Substances, EPA, Washington, DC.

FDA (1965). Illustrated Guide for Grading Eye Irritation by Hazardous Substances, FDA, Washington, DC.

FEDERAL HAZARDOUS SUBSTANCES ACT (1964). File 21, CFR 13009-101.12. Test for Eye Irritants. Federal Register.

FINKEL, A.J. (1983). Hamilton and Hardy's Industrial Toxicology, 4th Ed. John Wright PSG Inc., Boston.

FRAZIER, J.M., GAD, S.C., GOLDBERG, A.M. and MCCULLEY, J.P. (1987). A Critical Evaluation of Alternatives to Acute Ocular Irritation Testing. Mary Ann Liebert, Inc., New York.

FREEBERG, F.E., GRIFFITH, J.F., BRUCE, R.D., and BAY, P.H.S. (1984). Correlation of animal test methods with human experience for household products. J. Toxicol., Cut. Ocular Toxicol. **1**:53-64.

FREEBERG, F.E., NIXON, G.A., REER, D.J., WEAVER, J.E., BRUCE, R.D., GRIFFITH, J.F. and SANDERS, L.W. (1986). Human and rabbit eye response to chemical insult. Fund, App. Toxicol. **7**:626-634.

FRIEDENWALD, J.S., HUGHES, W.F. and HERRMANN, H. (1944). Arch. Ophthalmology. **31**:279.

GAD, S.C. and CHENGELIS, C.P. (1988). Acute Toxicology. Telford Press, Caldwell, NJ.

GAD, S.C. (1988). Defining product safety information and testing requirement . In Handbook of Product Safety Evaluation (S.C. Gad, ed.), pp. 1-22. Marcel Dekker, New York.

GAD, S.C., WALSH, R.D. and DUNN, B.J. (1986). Correlation of ocular and dermal irritancy of industrial chemicals. J. Toxicol., Cut. and Ocular Toxicol. **5**:193-211.

GILMAN, M.R. (1982). Skin and eye testing in animals. In Principles and Methods of Toxicology (A.W. Hayes,ed.), pp. 209-222. Raven Press, New York.

GILMAN, M.R., JACKSON, E.M., CERVEN, D.R. and MORENO, M.T. (1983). Relationship between the primary dermal irritation index and ocular irritation. J. Toxicol., Cut. and Ocular Toxicol. **2**:107-117.

GLASS, L. (1975). Classification of biological networks by their qualitative dynamics. J. Theor. Biol. **54**:85-107.

GLOXHUBER, C.H. (1985). Modification of the Draize eye test for the safety testing of cosmetics. Fd. Chem. Toxic. **23**:187-188.

GORDON, A.D. (1981). Classification. Chapman and Hall, New York.

GORDON, V.C. and BERGMEN, H.C. (1986). EYTEX, An *In Vitro* Method for Evaluation of Optical Irritancy. National Testing Corporation Report, 26.

GOSSELIN, R.E., SMITH, R.P. and HODGE, H.C. (1984). Clinical Toxicology of Commercial Products, 5th Ed. William and Wilkins, Baltimore.

GRANT, W.M. (1974). Toxicology of the Eye, 2nd Ed., Voumes I and II. Charles C. Thomas, Springfield, IL.

GREEN, W.R., SULLIVAN, J.B., HEHIR, R.M., SCHARPF, L.F. and DICKINSON, A.M. (1978). A Systemic Comparison of Chemically Induced Eye Injury in the Albino Rabbit and the Rhesus Monkey. The Soap and Detergent Association, New York.

GRIFFITH, J.F., NIXON, G.A., BRUCE, R.D., REER, P.J. and BANNAN, E.A. (1980). Dose-response studies with chemical irritants in the albino rabbit eye as a basis for selecting optimum testing conditions for predicting hazard to the human eye. Tox. Appl. Pharmacol. **55**:501-513.

GUILLOT, J.P., GONNET, J.F., CLEMENT, C., CAILLARD, L. and TRAHAUT, R. (1982). Evaluation of the cutaneous-irritation potential of 56 compounds. Fd. Chem. Toxicol. **20**:563-572.

GUILLOT, J.P. GONNET, J.F., CLEMENT, C. CAILLARD, L. and TRAHAUT, R. (1982). Evaluation of the cutaneous-irritation potential of 56 compounds. Fd. Chem. Toxicol. **20**:573-582.

INTERAGENCY REGULATORY LIAISON GROUP (1981). Testing Standards and Guidelines Work Group Recommended Guidelines. Code of Federal Regulations. Revised Jan. 1, 1981, Title 16: Subchapter C - Federal Hazardous Substances Act, part 1500.42, 1981 (Test for Eye Irritants).

JACARUSO, R.B., BARLETT, M.A., CARSON, S. and TROMBETTA, L.D. (1985). Release of histamine from rat peritoneal cells *in vitro* as an index of irritational potential. J. Toxicol., Cut. Ocular Toxicol. **4**:39-48.

JACKSON, E.M. (1983). Industrial practices in safety testing. In Product Safety Evaluation.(A.M. Goldberg, ed.). Alternative Methods in Toxicology, Vol.1, pp. 51-65. Mary Ann Liebert, Inc., New York.

JACKSON, J. and RUTTY, R.A. (1985). Ocular tolerance assessment-tier policy. Fd. Chem. Toxicol. **23**:309-310.

JAYJOCK, M.A. and GAD, S.C. Hazard and risk assessment. In Handbook of Products Safety Evaluation. (S.C. Gad, ed.), pp. 558-628. Marcel Dekker, New York.

JUMBLATT, M.M. and NEUFELD, A.H. (1985). A tissue culture model of the human corneal epithelium. In *In Vitro* Toxicology (A.M. Goldberg, ed.). Alternative Methods in Toxicology, Vol. 3, pp. 391-404. Mary Ann Liebert, Inc., New York .

KEMP, R.V., MEREDITH, R.W.J., GAMBLE, S. and FROST, M. (1983). A rapid cell culture technique for assaying to toxicity of detergent based products *in vitro* as a possible screen for high irritants *in vivo*. Cytobios **36**:153-159.

KEMP, R.V. MEREDITH, R.W.J. and GAMBLE, S. (1985). Toxicity of commercial products on cells in suspension: A possible screen for the Draize eye irritation test. Fd. Chem. Toxicol. **23**:267-270.

LATVEN, A.R. and MOLITOR, N. (1939). Comparison of the toxic, hypnotic and irritating properties of 8 organic solvents. J. Pharm. Exptl. Ther. **65**:89-94.

LEIGHTON, J., NASSAUER, J., TCHAO, R. and VERDONE, J. (1983). Development of a Procedure Using the Chick Egg as an Alternative to the Draize Rabbit Test. In Product Safety Evaluation (A.M. Goldberg, ed.), Alternative Methods in Toxicology, Vol. 1, pp. 165-177. Mary Ann Liebert, Inc., New York.

LUEPKE, N.P. (1981). Hen's egg choriollantoic membrane test for irritation potential. Fd. Chem. Toxicol. **23**:287-291.

MACKINSON, F. (1981). National Institute for Occupational Health and Safety/Occupational Safety and Health Administration (1981). Occupational Health Guidelines for Chemical Hazards. Department of Health and Human Services (NIOSH)/Department of Labor (OSHA) DHHS No. 81-123, Government Printing Office, Washington, DC.

MANN, I. and PULLINGER, D.B. (1942). A Study of mustard gas lesions of the eyes of rabbits and men. Proc. R. Soc. Med. **35**:229-244.

MARZULLI, F.N. and RUGLES, D.I. (1973). Rabbit eye irritation test: Collaborative study. J. Assoc. Off. Anal. Chem. **56**:905:914.

MAURICE, D. and SINGH, T. (1986). A permeability test for acute corneal toxicity. Toxicol. Letters **31**:125-130.

McCALLY, A.W., FARMER, A.G. and LOOMIS, E.C. (1933). Corneal Ulceration Following Use of Lash Lure. J. Amer. Med. Assoc. **101**:1560-1561.

McDONALD, T.O., SEABAUGH, V., SHADDUCK, J.A. and ADELHAUSER, H.F. (1983). Eye irritation In Dermatotoxicology (F.N. Marzulli and H.I. Maibach, eds.), pp. 556-610. Hemisphere Publishing, New York.

MCLAUGHLIN, R.S. (1946). Chemical burns of the human cornea. Am. J. Ophthalmol. 29:1355-1362.

MUIR, C.K. (1984). A simple method to assess surfactant-induced bovine corneal opacity *in vitro*: Preliminary findings. Toxicol. Letters **23**:199-203.

MUIR, C.K., FLOWER, C. and VAN ABBE, N.J. (1983). A novel approach to the search for *in vitro* alternatives to *in vivo* eye irritancy testing. Toxicol. Letters **18**:1-5.

MURPHY, J.C., OSTERBERG, R.E., SEABAUGH, V.M. and BIERBOWER (1982). Ocular irritance to various pHs of acids and bases with and without irrigation. Toxicology **23**:281-291.

NATIONAL ACADEMY OF SCIENCE (NAS) (1977). Principles and Procedures for Evaluating the Toxicity of Household Substances, pp. 41-59. NAS Publication 1138, Washington, D.C.

NATIONAL INSTITUTE OF OCCUPATIONAL SAFETY AND HEALTH (1984). Registry of Toxic Effects of Chemical Substances, 11th Ed., Volumes 1-3. Department of Health and Human Services DHHS No. 83-107, 1983 and RTECS Supplement DHHS 84-101. Washington, D.C.

NATIONAL INSTITUTE FOR OCCUPATIONAL SAFETY AND HEALTH, NIOSH Criteria for a Recommended Standard for Occupational Exposure. Department of Health, Education and Welfare. Cincinnati, OH.

NATIONAL INSTITUTE FOR OCCUPATIONAL SAFETY AND HEALTH. NIOSH Current Intelligence Bulletins. Department of Health, Education and Welfare. Cincinnati, OH.

NATIONAL LIBRARY OF MEDICINE, Office of Inquiries and Publications Management, 8600 Rockville Pike, Bethesda, MD 20209.

NORTH-ROOT, H., YACKOVICH, DEMETRULIAS, F.J., GUCULA, J. and HEINZE, J.E. (1982). Evaluation of an *in vitro* cell toxicity test using rabbit corneal cells to predict the eye irritation potential of surfactants. Toxicol. Letters **14**:207-212.

OLIVER, G.J.A. and PEMBERTON, N.A. (1985). An *in vitro* epidermal slice technique for identifying chemicals with potential for severe cutaneous effects. Fd. Chem. Toxicol. **23**:229-232.

ORGANIZATION FOR ECONOMIC COOPERATION AND DEVELOPMENT (1981). OECD Guidelines for Testing of Chemicals, Sect. 404, Acute Dermal Irritation/Corrosion, Paris.

PARKER, C.M. (1987). Available toxicology information source and their use. In Handbook of Product Safety Evaluation (S.C. Gad, ed.), pp. 23-41. Marcel Dekker, New York.

PROCTOR, N.H. and HUGHES, J.P. (1978). Chemical Hazards of the Workplace. J.B. Lippincott, Philadelphia.

REINHARDT, C.A., PELLI, D.A. and ZBINDEN, G. (1985). Interpretation of cell toxicity data for the estimation of potential irritation. Fd. Chem. Toxicol. **23**:247-252.

REINHARDT, C.A. and SCHLATTER, C.H. (1985). Acute irritation tests in risk assessment. Fd. Chem. Toxicol. **23**:145-148.

SAX, N.I. (1985). Dangerous Properties of Industrial Materials. 6th Ed. Van Nostrand Reinhold, New York.

SCAIFE, M.C. (1982). An investigation of detergent action on *in vitro* and possible correlation with *in vivo* data. Internat. J. Cosm. Sci. **4**:179-193.

SELLING, J. and EKWALL, B. (1985). Screening for eye irritancy using cultured Hela Cells. Xenobiotica **15**:713-717.

SHADDUCK, J.A., EVERITT, J. and BAY, P. (1985). Use of *in vitro* cytotoxicity to rank ocular irritation of six surfactants. In *In Vitro* Toxicology. (A.M. Goldberg, ed.). Alternative Methods in Toxicology, Vol. 3 A, pp. 641-649. Mary Ann Liebert, Inc., New York.

SHADDUCK, J.A., RENDER, J., EVERITT, J., MECOOLI, R.A. and ESSEX-SHOPSIS, C. and ENG, B. (1985). Uridine uptake and cell growth cytotoxicity tests: Comparison, applications and mechanistic studies. J. Cell Biol. **101**:87a.

SHOPSIS, C. and SATHE, A. (1984). Uridine uptake inhibition as a cytotoxicity test: Correlation with the Draize test. Toxicology **29**:195-206.

SILVERMAN, J. (1983). Preliminary findings on the use of protozoa (*Tetrahymena thermophila*) as models for ocular irritation testing in rabbits. Lab. Animal Sci. **33**:55-59.

SIMONS, P.J. (1981). An alternative to the Draize test. In Use of Alternatives in Drug Research (A.N. Rowan and C.J. Stratmann, Eds.). MacMillan Press, Ltd., London.

SITTIG, M. (1981). Handbook of Toxic and Hazardous Chemicals. Noyes Park Ridge, NJ.

SORLIE, D. (1987). An Approach to validation: Comparison of six materials in three tests. *In Vitro* Toxicology-Approaches to Validation. Alternative Methods in Toxicology, Vol. 5. Mary Ann Liebert, Inc., New York.

SWANSTON, D.W. (1985). Assessment of the validity of animal techniques in eye irritation testing. Fd. Chem. Toxicol. **23**:169-173.

TALSMA, D.M., LEACH, C.L., HATOUM, N.S., GIBBONS, R.D., ROGER, J.C. and GARVIN, P.J. (1988). Reducing the number of rabbits in the Draize eye irritancy test: A statistical analysis of 155 studies conducted over 6 years. Fund. Appl. Toxicol. **10**:146-153.

WALKER, A.P. (1985). A more realistic animal technique for predicting human eye responses. Fd. Chem. Toxicol. **23**:175-178.

WEIL, C.S. and SCALA, R.A. (1971). Study of intra- and interlaboratory variability in the results of rabbit eye and skin irritation tests. Toxicol. Appl. Pharmacol. **19**:276-360.

WETERINGS, P.J.J.M. and VAN ERP, Y.H.M. (1987). Validation of the Becam assay - an eye irritancy screening test. In *In Vitro* Toxicology: Approaches to Validation (A.M. Goldberg, ed.), pp. 515-521. Mary Ann Liebert, Inc., New York.

WEXLER, P. (1987). Information Resources in Toxicology, 2nd Ed. Elsevier, New York.

WILLIAMS, S.J. (1984). Prediction of ocular irritancy potential from dermal irritation test results. Fd. Chem. Toxicol. **2**:157-161.

WILLIAMS, S.J., GRAEPEL, G.J. and KENNEDY, G.L. (1982). Evaluation of ocular irritancy potential: Intralaboratory variability and effect of dosage volume. Toxicol. Letters **12**:235-241.
WINDHOLZ, M. (1983). The Merck Index, 10th Ed. Merck and Company, Inc., Rahway, NJ.

ANIMAL RIGHTS AND MODERN TOXICOLOGY

LEONARD RACK AND HENRY SPIRA

Animal Rights
New York, New York

"Pain and suffering are bad and should be prevented or minimized, irrespective of the race, sex, or species of the being that suffers....To discriminate against beings solely on account of their species is a form of prejudice, immoral and indefensible...." Peter Singer, in *Animal Liberation* (1975), the manifesto of the animal rights movement.

"Do [animals] feel fear? Locked in a laboratory, do they mourn their freedom? Do they hear the footsteps in the corridor and wonder whose cage they will stop at this time?" "Once, it would have been inconceivable to entertain these questions seriously....Today they are central to one of the fastest-growing causes in America....animal rights." *Newsweek*, May 23, 1988.

Ten years ago, this monograph would not have been possible. The publication in this country of such a record of collaboration of internationally renowned toxicologists in alternative efforts signals a historic shift in sentiment and outlook.

Where formerly the goals of animal welfare and the goals of creative science appeared diametrically opposed, both scientists and the public are now realizing that they can convert walls into bridges by joining forces in promoting shared goals of better science, efficiency, economy and humanity, and that the collaborative joining of forces can only enhance progress along all these axes.

We hope in this chapter to demonstrate some of the bases for this bridge-building. Much of this book can be seen as presenting the nuts, bolts, struts and girders for this connection. We feel that our recent rapid progress stems from the confluence of two novel currents in modern history.

The first is the development of a series of rights movements including civil rights, women's rights and animal rights, each gaining clarity and courage from the successes of their predecessors. Only fairly recently has it been generally accepted that all humans, regardless of sex, race or popularity, are entitled to have their interests

---

1. Address correspondence to: Mr. Henry Spira, Animal Rights, P.O. Box 214, Planetarium Station, New York, NY 10024.

2. Key words: animal rights, reduction, refinement, replacement.

3. Abbreviations: ASTM, American Society of Testing and Materials; CTFA, Cosmetic, Toiletry and Fragrance Association; NSMR, National Society for Medical Research; NTP, National Toxicology Program; PMA, Pharmaceutical Manufacturers Association.

respected. Once all humans have been included in our "expanding circle of concern," consistency mandates that we work to include other species, non-human animals, who, like you and me, seek to avoid pain and attempt to get a little pleasure out of life. As Jeremy Bentham posed the issue more than 200 years ago, "The question is not, Can they reason? nor Can they talk? but, Can they *suffer?*"

The other current is the spectacular exponential development of modern science, with the flow in the direction of the microscopic, sub-microscopic and molecular. This developing technology buttresses our hope that people's increasingly assertive humane sympathies can find expression in innovative, seminal and usable scientific discoveries. In the real world, given our current technology and understanding, some organisms will be harmed to help others. Still, we can marshall serious energies to reduce pain and suffering as much and as rapidly as possible.

What is particularly encouraging is that scientists are now recognizing that, in the process of looking for alternatives, they can gain fundamental and thus highly beneficial scientific understandings and at the same time gratify deep humane impulses.

We wish to discuss the past, present and possible future of these flows. We will outline past issues, including the accelerating development of the past ten years. We shall then review briefly some current "cooking soups" that were discussed in other contexts in earlier chapters. We shall speculate about a future in which the search for alternatives will become a regularly accepted way of doing business in advancing a progressively more elegant and non-intrusive science. Hopefully, the intrinsic excitement of these flows will resonate with readers' intellectual/ethical curiosity and commitment.

PAST AS PROLOGUE

In the old days, biological scientists and animal protectionists were usually to be found at each other's throats, each screaming that the other was immoral. This deplorable state of affairs, dependent on a black-and-white, saints-and-sinners way of looking at the issues, ruled the past century and did no good to anyone, including the animals.

Fortunately, early in the century, a small but rapidly growing cadre of visionary philosopher/scientists emerged. They conceived the possibility that the goals of science and of the animal protection movement need not be contradictory, that difficult as the idea might at first appear, humane science would be better science.

Individuals working within this framework produced a series of suggestions as to what was doable. In 1957, Charles W. Hume, founder of the Universities Federation for Animal Welfare, in a 1957 *Lancet* article, "The Strategy and Tactics of Experimentation," suggested that toxicity testing could dispense with the LD_{50}, a suggestion which was later to be amplified by Gerhard Zbinden, the illustrious contributor of the first chapter in this volume.

Two years later, W.M.S. Russell and R.L. Burch published their ground-breaking volume, "The Principles of Humane Experimental Technique" (Methuen & Co., London), the "bible" of the alternatives movement. In it, they discussed alternatives to the Draize test, which was developed in the early 1940's, and the LD_{50}, developed in 1927. They also suggested multiple ingenious methods, e.g., naturalistic methods for the study of tranquilizers and analgesics, for realization of the project they christened the "three R's": Reduction of numbers of animals used, Replacement of animals with alternatives, Refinement of methods to decrease their pain and distress. Throughout, they emphasized that increasingly humane scientific methods, introducing fewer artifacts, would produce better science.

In 1978, David Smyth, the late head of the British Research Defense Society, published "Alternatives to Animal Experiments" (Scolar Press, London), which explored potential alternatives in biology. As Russell and Burch had done, Smyth attempted the difficult task of defining where alternatives were possible versus areas in which animal use, at the time, appeared essential. He specifically suggested tissue culture as an alternative to the Draize eye irritation test, a suggestion that was first taken up and then temporarily forgotten, evidently buried under the weight of the then-current traditional views.

All of these various suggestions gradually percolated about but finally came to critical mass within the past decade and were adopted by the animal protection movement in specific campaigns.

THE DRAIZE TEST

Smyth had proposed replacement of the Draize both because it clearly caused suffering and because he felt that the development of an alternative, e.g., with tissue culture, should not present any major scientific problems. On study of the research materials available, we concurred and decided to approach corporations that used Draize testing, hoping to gain their collaboration in seeking an alternative. We began by attempting discussions with a cosmetics industry leader, Revlon.

At first, Revlon refused to consider the potential of alternatives, perhaps "considering the source." But after more than two years of protests by our coalition of animal protectionists against the use of the Draize, Revlon responded by funding a group of researchers at Rockefeller University to seek cell biological and other humane alternatives to the test, thus institutionalizing and carrying forward the seminal suggestions of Smyth and of other British scientists. The Rockefeller group generated new ideas and findings and spawned similar major programs in West Germany and Switzerland.

This initiative by the biomedical-research-industrial complex was the "big bang" needed by the alternatives movement, an immense leap forward in establishing the legitimacy and promise of the search for alternatives.

As part of this initial thrust, the idea of giving alternatives a fair shake was furthered significantly by the trailblazing activities of a number of corporate toxicologists, Ted Brenner, John Corbett, Pam Danneman, Yale Gressel, Jack Griffith, Myron Mehlman, Jim Russo, Bob Scala, Janice Teal, Alex Vongries, John Yam; government scientists, Gary Ellis, Ted Farber, John Moore, Gary Flamm, Victor Morgenroth, David Rall; and science writers, Jeannie Blake, Mary Brevnik, Ron Dagani, Susan Fowler, Jane Gregory, Cathy Heinze, Constance Holden, Rex Rhein, Helen Smith, Nicholas Wade, Jonathan Weiner among others.

This momentum and our negotiations with Avon, Bristol-Myers, Estée Lauder, and other well-known companies created the Center for Alternatives to Animal Testing at Johns Hopkins. From the program's inception, we urged development of new toxicologic methods, indicating both that a public increasingly concerned with animal protection desired change and that such change was now a good bet scientifically and economically.

The Johns Hopkins alternatives program distributed many small grants, piggybacking the search for alternatives on to massive research projects which were already in progress. This brought established researchers into the alternatives loop. In addition, symposia and publications encouraged the networking of scientists developing new methods for research and testing.

And now these research efforts are beginning to pay off. New techniques, some of which are mentioned earlier in this book, have been developed and some are now being validated in anticipation of practical application. Some leading corporations have already included eye irritation alternatives in their own labs. And federal agencies have changed their policies so that substances known to be irritants, such as lye, ammonia and oven cleaners, need not be retested in the eyes of rabbits.

Requirements are being harmonized so that data can be shared, and, as a result of sophisticated statistical studies, the suggested number of rabbits needed per test for other products has been reduced by one-half to one-third.

The Soap and Detergent Association and the Cosmetic, Toiletry and Fragrance Association, in cooperation with the regulatory sectors, are organizing projects to select the most promising non-animal alternative methods to the Draize, so that industry can, in a uniform manner, incorporate these alternatives into their standard testing procedures.

Finally, as a vastly improved interim measure, P&G has developed, pending validation of entirely non-animal testing, its "low-volume" test, which uses one-tenth the concentration of irritant. This test has been accepted by the American Society of Testing and Materials (ASTM) and P&G has found it to be more predictive of human experience than the conventional Draize.

It's likely that alternative methods can do as well or better than the Draize even now and can probably be developed toward much greater precision and accuracy.

THE LD$_{50}$ TEST

How, we asked ourselves, could the success of the "Rockefeller-Hopkins" campaign be used as an Archimedian fulcrum for leverage in moving the resistant, doubting world in the direction of Reduction, Replacement and Refinement? Keeping this in mind, we decided to focus next on the classic LD$_{50}$, the 61-year old toxicologic test we felt was most wasteful, one that a growing number of scientists questioned.

As early as 1957, at the height of acceptance of the LD$_{50}$ as the benchmark of toxicologic testing, Hume had suggested that it might be possible to choose some measurable effect of a drug, other than death, to test toxicity, and had wondered whether the extensive use of the LD$_{50}$ was a "hangover due to habit and custom."

In addition, in 1978, Smyth had questioned the rationale for the expanding use of the LD$_{50}$, indicating that Trevan, who developed the LD$_{50}$, was concerned not with the potential harm of unknown substances but with the standardization of substances in medical use that are poisonous in concentrations close to the beneficial range. Smyth had pointed out the contradiction that "a test for lethal toxicity is really being used as a test for non-lethal toxicity, or at least to give assurances about non-lethal toxicity"—that is, death is being used as a test for sickness.

Finally, in 1973, Dr. Gerhard Zbinden, a world leader in toxicology, challenging the rationale for the LD$_{50}$ test, had described it as "a ritual mass execution of animals." Again, in 1976, Dr. Zbinden had commented that most experts considered the routine LD$_{50}$ "a wasteful endeavor in which scientific inventiveness and common sense have been replaced by a thoughtless completion of senseless protocols" and had suggested that methods using more careful study of fewer animals would yield more useful information. In 1982, Zbinden had asserted that "Clinical experience shows that the LD$_{50}$ value determined in animals rarely bears a meaningful relation with the lethal dose in man." Zbinden suggested regulatory change from the classic LD$_{50}$ using 50 to 200 animals to range-finding tests using six to ten animals with careful observation.

Zbinden was not alone. At the Royal Society of London meeting of the Fund for the Replacement of Animals in Medical Experiments, sponsored by Ciba-Geigy in November, 1982, scientists from pharmaceutical companies, by a show of hands, voted 20 to one to abolish the LD$_{50}$. In addition, at a Bristol-Myers-sponsored meeting focusing on the LD$_{50}$ at Baltimore's Johns Hopkins Center for Alternatives, the participants concluded that alternatives—for example, range-finding—would "ensure public health while using as few as one-tenth the number of animals now used."

During this period, Procter & Gamble was urging the adoption of a new "up/down LD_{50}" method requiring one-fourth the number of animals, an alternative recently accepted by the ASTM.

The LD_{50} issue seemed to us to be the perfect example of "cultural lag," in which the spread of information in the right directions would lead to action. But, at this juncture, we needed the commitment of corporate scientific expertise towards replacement and reduction. So we contacted the Pharmaceutical Manufacturers Association (PMA) and a number of member companies and urged the corporations to promote alternatives in-house while encouraging the PMA to challenge the LD_{50} publicly. This initial effort, a collaboration with grassroots activist organizations, started the ball rolling.

On October 21, 1982, the PMA, representing 149 research-based US pharmaceutical companies, asserted that "neither the toxicologist nor the clinical pharmacologist needs a precise LD_{50} value" and that "regulatory requirements should accommodate this position." The PMA's position was seconded by the Cosmetic, Toiletry & Fragrance Association (CTFA) and by the Soap & Detergent Association (SDA).

Next, we contacted the National Society for Medical Research (NSMR), whereupon their Board of Directors unanimously approved a statement, which was adopted on December 14, 1982, that the "routine use of the quantitative LD_{50} is not now scientifically justified..." and Dr. David P. Rall, Director of the National Toxicology Program (NTP), wrote to us on March 3, 1983 saying that the classic LD_{50} "is now an anachronism....I do not think the LD_{50} test provides much useful information about the health hazards to humans... . The NTP does not use the LD_{50}."

The expression of the consensus included ten cover stories in major US science/industry publications and a letter from Congressman Bill Green (NY) signed by 73 other members of the U.S. Congress asking federal agencies to eliminate the LD_{50}. In response to the growing consensus within the science community, the Food & Drug Administration met on November 9, 1983 to review and clarify its policies. They emphasized that the classic LD_{50} is not required for regulatory purposes.

The consequences of these regulatory assertions were far-reaching. Surveys by our Coalition indicate an approximately 75% reduction over the past five years in the number of animals used in acute oral safety testing. The decrease was attributed to the use of "limit" and "range-finding" tests as well as data banks. And the results of a survey at a Food & Drug Administration center prompted the center's director, Dr. Gary Flamm, to comment, "These figures are encouraging signs, indicating the classic LD_{50} test is becoming a thing of the past."

Still, though much progress has been made towards eliminating the classic LD_{50}, in routine toxicity studies much still remains to be done. Given the scientific consensus in favor of change away from the routine use of the test, it appears that the only remaining roadblock is that inertia which expectedly stems from people's fear of change, particularly in issues of safety. But we feel that a complete victory over the

LD$_{50}$ is possible, will not endanger safety, and will be of enormous importance since it will save animals from needless and painful poisoning, and will encourage the pattern of reassessment of traditional testing.

THE EXPANDING LOOP/THE PERCOLATING PRESENT

Progress toward phasing down the classic LD$_{50}$ and Draize tests has been much faster than expected. Ten years ago, replacing these tests appeared overwhelmingly difficult. But as events developed, the scientific clarity of the objections to these tests and the evident goodwill of a number of corporations and governmental agencies have, in combination, led to superbly encouraging results.

At each step, noting the way in which wasteful practices had become unquestioned givens, our coalitions have stressed the need for institutional structural reviews and ongoing, regular critical self-evaluation on the part of all organizations that use or promote the use of animals. We feel that such self-critical practice follows the best self-questioning tradition of science. A self-questioning strategy that we have suggested is "zero-based" animal use, an adaptation of zero-based budgeting. In zero-based budgeting, an entire budget is examined and alternatives evaluated as if the program were being prepared for the first time, starting from zero. This may be contrasted with incremental budgeting, where the previous year's budget is the baseline, and increments are simply added on. The successes of the Draize and LD$_{50}$ enterprises embolden us to believe that the zero-based concept can be fruitfully incorporated into ongoing efforts to replace animals in testing.

In line with the zero-based concept, we have suggested to those who use animals the following initiatives:

- To energetically promote the development, validation and implementation of batteries of alternatives for specific product categories.
- To make an internal commitment to promote reduction, replacement and refinement, and to generate an annual, public report of accomplishments and long-term plans.
- To develop or commission feasibility studies or White Papers on promising public policy, research, development, and implementation opportunities.
- To attend to the crucial importance of ongoing and increasing education of laboratory personnel in alternative methods.

But the animal movement has not in isolation been dreaming up ways to "think alternatives." Over the past six years, such major corporations as Avon, Bristol-Myers, Colgate, Hoffmann-La Roche, Mobil and Procter & Gamble have instituted procedural changes comprising many of the above initiatives.

- One recent corporate initiative, which we believe will have far-reaching effect, is a joint undertaking by leading toxicologists Myron A. Mehlman from Mobil, Emil

A. Pfitzer from Hoffmann-La Roche and Robert A. Scala from Exxon. Earlier this year, they issued an invitation to all major industrial toxicology labs to share any procedures which have immediate practical application. To speed this task along, they contracted with an impartial industry consultant to coordinate the identification and sharing of viable alternatives. The technology transfer will be handled so that proprietary information will not be threatened, thus increasing potential participation in the project.

- Procter & Gamble has developed an alternative to the classic LD_{50} and a modified Draize test, both of which were recently accepted by the American Society for Testing and Materials. P&G is now seeking non-animal tests for birth defects, cancer-causing effects, lung damage, skin irritation, skin allergy, eye irritation and respiratory allergy. On the public policy front, P&G continues to energetically promote the implementation of alternatives through forums, publications and presentations directed to the industrial, academic and regulatory sectors.

- Mobil Corporation has developed a computerized system which permits 95-98% of new formulations to be approved without new animal testing. In addition, Mobil has replaced much of its traditional chronic skin cancer testing on animals with the Mobil Modified Ames bacterial test. At Mobil alone, this alternative is saving 30,000 animals per year.

- Colgate-Palmolive has also reduced animal use by 80% over the past 6 years. Colgate holds regular meetings throughout the corporate structure to promote and share alternative methods, and has established an "Alternatives Research" post-doctorate fellowship program in association with the Society of Toxicology. Colgate has developed potential alternatives in the company's own facilities, including the Chorioallantoic Membrane Assay [CAM] test, the skin cell culture assay and the yeast cell phototoxicity test.

- Avon has reduced its use of animals by 72% over the past six years, in part through the use of a computer system that allows their researchers to approve more than 90% of all new formulas without conducting additional animal tests. The company is also funding a three-year contact allergy testing project, which, because of recent advances in immunology, Avon researchers feel will be an area in which alternatives can rapidly be implemented.

Activity is also increasing on the federal research and regulatory fronts. The National Toxicology Program (NTP), under the leadership of David P. Rall, M.D., is making significant strides towards replacing and reducing the use of animals through a program aimed at developing and validating new methods of identifying environmental health hazards. Currently (FY 88), the NTP is allocating $17.7 million of its $79 million annual budget (22%) towards this program. In a recent conference on Public Health Service policy, Dr. Rall said, "We must aggressively continue to expand our efforts to discover new methods. Whenever the science allows, we need to substitute with approaches that use the fewest animals possible, or that eliminate the need for animals altogether. We cannot, however, dictate specific methods to the laboratory scientists. These must be allowed to evolve as an integral part of his or her line of investigation."

PREVISION OF THINGS FUTURE

The public and political context of animal rights will play an important role in determining the direction and success of animal rights concerns in toxicology proper. Rightly or wrongly, regulatory decisions as well as funding are strongly influenced by public and political response. Thus, our prospective activities include surveys of public attitudes, intensified educational efforts, influence against frivolous use of animals in the educational process, and a challenge of current factory farming practices.

All of the percolating flows described, the "cooking soups" of the present, need to be crystallized into definite and accepted procedures. We have described some of the ongoing efforts to accomplish this desirable end and confidently expect success in the near future. What might we outline as possibilities for the larger future?

We, as well as others, have suggested consensus conferences involving toxicologists, government regulators internationally, the product liability sector, the academic community and consumer groups. Toxicologists can play a key role in the process as scientific educators and leaders.

All local endeavors will require international consensus. Otherwise, products which are sold internationally will be tested by the guidelines of the country with the most restrictive, cumbersome regulations. We anticipate that in this area the universal scientific spirit will prevail and that new, more efficient methodologies will be recognized as such and pressed into service.

Accelerating scientific interest, activity and accomplishment in the alternatives area bode well for the future. The number of publications, journals and books currently devoted to alternatives is increasing geometrically. Recent books include 1) "Alternatives to Animal Use in Research, Testing and Education" by the U.S. Congress' Office of Technology Assessment (OTA), which has had an immediate, practical impact on OTA staff developing expertise which they have, in turn, shared with Congressional staffers, 2) Andrew Rowan's "Of Mice, Models, and Men—A Critical Evaluation of Animal Research," and 3) Mary Ann Liebert's series of books Alternative Methods in Toxicology.

Current journals about alternatives, many begun in the explosive developments of the past few years, include:

- The 14-year old *Alternatives to Laboratory Animals* (ATLA), the scientific journal of The Fund for the Replacement of Animals in Medical Experiments (FRAME), edited by Michael Balls. ATLA was the pioneer alternatives journal.

FRAME, Eastgate House, 34 Stoney St., Nottingham, Great Britain NG1 1NB; (0602) 584-6740.

- *Cell Biology and Toxicology*, edited by Gary Williams, launched in 1984. Princeton Scientific Publishing Co., Inc., P.O. Box 2155, Princeton, NJ 08543; (609) 683-4750.
- *Toxicology and Industrial Health*, edited by Jim R. Withey, launched in 1985. Publishes papers on alternatives in pharmacology, cell biology and tissue culture. Princeton Scientific Publishing Co., Inc., P.O. Box 2155, Princeton, NJ 08543; (609) 683-4750.
- *In-Vitro Toxicology*, launched in 1986, edited by David Brusick. Mary Ann Liebert Inc., 1651 Third Ave., NYC 10128; (212) 289-2300.
- *Molecular Toxicology*, launched in 1987, edited by Stanley Scher. Harper & Row, 1010 Vermont Ave. NW, Washington, DC 20005; (202) 783-3958.
- *Toxicology in Vitro*, an international journal published in association with the British Industrial Biological Research Association (BIBRA), launched in 1987, edited by I.F.H. Purchase and G.C. Hard. Pergamon Journals Inc., Maxwell House, Fairview Pk., Elmsford, NY 10523; (914) 592-7700.

Visionary biology/high-tech entrepreneurs have begun to realize the great promise in alternatives:

- Organogenesis, a biochemical company, is developing living tissues and organs, including a Living Skin Equivalent, from human cells and tissue matrix molecules. An initial focus is the development of test systems to assay the toxicity of substances. Organogenesis Inc., 83 Rogers St., Cambridge, MA 02142, (617) 577-1717.
- The National Testing Corporation (NTC) has developed an alternative to the Draize procedure called Eytex. It turns cloudy when mixed with substances that would produce eye irritation, and remains clear in the presence of non-irritants. NTC says Eytex has a 96% correlation with the Draize. NTC, 888 Research Dr., Palm Springs, CA 92262, (619) 323-8474.
- Clonetics Corporation produces commercially available strains of normal human skin cells from the upper surface of the skin, and has developed seven test systems using this culture. The company reports that 125 companies and academic researchers now use the cells. Clonetics Corp., 9620 Chesapeake Dr., San Diego, CA 92123, (619) 541-0086.

In line with this ferment in the private sector, we have suggested that the National Institutes of Health (NIH), the organizational nerve-center of U.S. biologic research, establish a series of cell technology centers around the country that would serve as resources and stimulation for progress in cellular and molecular biology/toxicology.

In a scant decade, a whole new discipline, *in vitro* toxicology, has taken shape, propelled by the scientific enthusiasm and excitement, generated by people's discussions and discoveries in seeking alternatives to traditional animal testing methods. We have detailed some of the major steps along the way and outlined some of the plans for the future.

The growing realization that "everyone wins" by these researches and practices will make it increasingly difficult for people to conceive of doing without them. The search for alternatives will become integrally part of the traditional mainstream, a part of everyone's modus operandi, a familiar tool in the tool box of the advancement of learning, in and out of universities, in and out of industry, wherever people look for answers to questions in biology.

UTILITY OF SHORT-TERM TESTS FOR GENETIC TOXICITY

DAVID M. DeMARINI,[a] JOELLEN LEWTAS,[a] AND HERMAN E. BROCKMAN[b]

By definition, short-term tests (STTs) for genetic toxicity detect genotoxic agents, not carcinogens specifically. However, there is sufficient evidence, based on mechanistic considerations alone, to say that genotoxic agents are potential carcinogens. STTs have high statistical power, are almost always replicated, can be performed rather easily under various sets of experimental conditions, are relatively inexpensive, and detect a variety of endpoints relevant to carcinogenesis. In addition, several STTs have shown considerable utility in evaluating the genotoxic effects of real-world, environmental complex mixtures as well as the antimutagenic effects of various pure compounds and complex mixtures. STTs are likely to continue to be refined, resulting in STTs that are increasingly more relevant to human mutation and disease. Their utility should not be judged solely against the questionable standard of a rodent carcinogenicity assay.

INTRODUCTION

Over 200 short-term tests (STTs) are now developed (Waters et al., 1988b); and more, no doubt, will be developed. This rich evolution of short-term tests, which has occurred since the development of the first STT by Muller (1927), has led to the recognition that the detection of genotoxic agents by means of STTs is important in its own right, quite apart from the detection of potential carcinogens. For example, there is now evidence that genotoxic agents may play an important role in the cause and/or progression of human diseases other than cancer. Hartman (1983) and Hartman and Morgan (1985) have reviewed the evidence that somatic mutations initiate focal lesions, including senile cataracts, metaplasias, and fibrous atherosclerotic plaques. Recently, Penn et al. (1986) have reported additional support for the role of somatic mutation in atherosclerosis by finding evidence for a transforming gene in human

[a]Genetic Bioassay Branch, Genetic Toxicology Division, U.S. Environmental Protection Agency, Research Triangle Park, NC 27711.
[b]Department of Biological Sciences, Illinois State University, Normal, IL 61761.

This manuscript has been reviewed by the Health Effects Research Laboratory, U.S. Environmental Protection Agency, and approved for publication. Approval does not signify that the contents necessarily reflect the views and policies of the Agency, nor does mention of trade names or commercial products constitute endorsement or recommendation for use.

atherosclerotic plaque DNA. Germ-cell mutations are also of obvious importance for certain human diseases (Crow, 1986).

Despite the abundant evidence for the utility of STTs in detecting genotoxic pure compounds (Rosenkranz, 1988) as well as genotoxic complex mixtures (DeMarini, 1989; Lewtas, 1989), a recent report by Tennant et al. (1987) has questioned the utility of STTs and of genetic toxicology itself. Their data led them to conclude that "No single *in vitro* STT adequately anticipates the diverse mechanisms of carcinogenesis; and, more important, the advantage of a battery of *in vitro* STTs is not supported by results of the present study. If current *in vitro* STTs are expected to replace long-term rodent studies for the identification of chemical carcinogens, then that expectation should be abandoned." On the other hand, the authors expressed support for the continued use of STTs by stating that "...because of health concerns apart from cancer, it seems prudent not to dismiss as significant the *in vitro* mutagenicity of the noncarcinogens. STTs...continue to offer an economical, rapid, and dependable means to detect genotoxic chemicals."

This mixed message of Tennant et al. (1987) has resulted in confusion and uncertainty regarding the role of STTs (Brusick, 1988); and the concerns raised by Tennant et al. (1987) have been addressed recently by various authors (Ashby, 1988; Ashby and Tennant, 1988; Bridges, 1988; Brockman and DeMarini, 1988; Heddle, 1988; ICPEMC, 1988; Sugimura, 1988; Trosko, 1988). In the present paper, we discuss some of the issues that pertain to the utility of STTs [see Brockman and DeMarini (1988) for a more detailed account of this topic]. In particular, we discuss: (1) concordance between carcinogenicity results in rats and mice and results in STTs, as well as concordance between the two rodents; (2) the influence of chemical class on sensitivity and specificity; (3) the utility of STTs and rodents for detecting human carcinogens; (4) the disadvantages of standardized protocols; (5) the importance of replicate experiments; (6) genotoxic noncarcinogens and nongenotoxic carcinogens; and (7) the utility of STTs for evaluating complex environmental mixtures and for detecting antimutagens.

CONCORDANCE BETWEEN RODENTS AND STTs, AND BETWEEN THE TWO RODENTS

When Tennant et al. (1987) compared STT results against mouse and rat carcinogenicity results for 74 chemicals, they concluded that, based on concordance, each STT (or a battery of all four STTs) performed about equally well ($\sim$ 60% concordance). Their data produced a similar concordance (67%) between rat and mouse carcinogenicity. This relatively low concordance between rat and mouse carcinogenicity results is not surprising. The strains of the two rodent species used exhibited different background tumor incidences at different sites, and different responses to the same chemical (Haseman, 1983). It is precisely for these reasons that different species are used in the rodent carcinogenicity assay.

What, perhaps, is unexpected is that the mouse (or rat) is no better than the STTs at identifying rat (or mouse) carcinogens or noncarcinogens. This is especially interesting considering the substantial differences between a bacterium (Salmonella) and a rodent, and the substantial similarities between a rat and a mouse. This relatively low concordance between rat and mouse carcinogenicity results has been noted by others (Lijinsky, 1988; McGregor, 1987). However, Ashby (1988) has argued that, based on the data of Tennant et al. (1987), the overall values for the cross-sensitivity between species are not critical for the detection of nongenotoxic carcinogens.

The fact that many carcinogens exhibit different carcinogenic effects in different species (or strains) is now well documented (Haseman, 1983; Nesnow et al., 1987; Tennant et al., 1987). As pointed out by Bridges (1986, 1988) and restated by Sobels (1987), "...carcinogenicity is expressed to a different extent in different species of rodents, so that bio-assay results in only two rodent species are likely to underestimate the proportion of chemicals with carcinogenic potential." This variation in response to a chemical among different species (or strains) complicates extrapolation not only from STTs to rodents, and from one rodent to another, but also from rodents to humans (Brusick, 1983; Roe, 1987).

The inappropriateness of rodent carcinogenicity assays as currently performed has been examined by Roe (1987), who notes that "There can be no sense in testing chemicals for carcinogenicity in rats maintained under conditions such that 50-100% of them [the control animals] develop pituitary and mammary tumors, etc. There is no identifiable population of humans for which such rats could constitute a model." The implications of these observations for risk assessment have been noted by Bridges (1986).

INFLUENCE OF CHEMICAL CLASS ON SENSITIVITY AND SPECIFICITY

The role of chemical class was not explored by Tennant et al. (1987) because the data base was too small to permit such an analysis. However, the influence of chemical class on sensitivity and specificity has been recognized for more than 12 years (McCann and Ames, 1976) and has been discussed recently in detail (Claxton, 1988; Ray et al., 1987; Zeiger, 1987). Because relatively large numbers of chemicals of various chemical classes have been tested in Salmonella, the role of chemical class can best be examined using the Salmonella data base.

The general conclusion that has emerged from such analyses is that sensitivity and specificity are greatly influenced by chemical class, and that the Salmonella assay is best used to identify rodent carcinogens and noncarcinogens when the results are interpreted within the context of chemical class. For example, Salmonella has a high sensitivity (85%) but low specificity (36%) for nitrogen-containing organics; conversely, it has a low sensitivity (63%) but high specificity (91%) for halogenated organics

(Claxton et al., 1988). Thus, calculations of overall sensitivity and specificity should consider chemical class.

UTILITY OF STTs AND RODENTS FOR DETECTING HUMAN CARCINOGENS

Rodent carcinogenicity assays are performed with the implied (if not the expressed) purpose of providing some insight into whether a particular chemical is a potential human carcinogen. Wilbourn et al. (1986) have calculated an 84% sensitivity value for rodent carcinogenicity results for the chemicals, groups of chemicals, and complex mixtures for which sufficient or limited evidence has been established by IARC for carcinogenicity to humans (IARC, 1982). Shelby (1988) reported a sensitivity value of 77% for the Salmonella assay among 22 of IARC's Group I chemicals (or groups of chemicals), which are designated as causally associated with cancer in humans (IARC, 1982). Of these, 91% were positive in one or both of the Salmonella and rodent bone marrow cytogenetic assays (Shelby, 1988). Thus, the sensitivities of STTs (and of laboratory animal carcinogenicity assays) for detecting human carcinogens are high. For these human carcinogens, there is no indication that laboratory animal carcinogenicity assays are superior to STTs in detecting human carcinogens. The same conclusion was reached by Brusick (1983) based on a similar analysis.

Further support for the utility of STTs for detecting human carcinogens has been provided by Garrett et al. (1984). Their detailed analyses of the quantitative and qualitative genotoxic activities of 24 known or suspected human carcinogens showed that chemically similar carcinogens produced similar types of genotoxic activities. Furthermore, they identified certain STTs that were more appropriate than others for detecting the genotoxicity of some classes of human carcinogens. In this regard, Shelby (1988) has shown recently that just two STTs, Salmonella and rodent bone marrow cytogenetic assays, detected 91% of a set of human carcinogens. Thus, STTs appear to be as useful as laboratory animal carcinogenicity assays for detecting either human or laboratory animal carcinogens.

DISADVANTAGES OF STANDARDIZED PROTOCOLS

The STT and carcinogenicity results generated and analyzed by Tennant et al. (1987) for 73 chemicals is unique in that all of the data were obtained by using standardized protocols. Although the advantages of using standardized protocols are clear, such protocols also pose disadvantages. It is obvious that the result of a particular experiment was obtained for the set of conditions under which that particular experiment was performed. However, under some other set of experimental conditions, the result may be different. The importance of testing under more than one set of conditions has been discussed in detail by Roe (1987) and is illustrated dramatically for benzene.

Numerous epidemiological studies indicated that benzene was a human carcinogen;

yet, from 1932 until recently, 14 carcinogenicity studies in laboratory animals failed to find evidence that benzene was a carcinogen (Huff et al., 1989). Likewise, most of the initial studies of the genotoxicity of benzene were also negative (Huff et al., 1989). Because of the compelling epidemiological data, efforts to demonstrate the carcinogenicity and genotoxicity of benzene were not abandoned. Finally, under certain test conditions (2-year gavage in rodents and in vivo cytogenetics in rodent bone marrow), benzene was clearly demonstrated to be a rodent carcinogen and genotoxicant (Huff et al., 1989). In the absence of the driving force of epidemiological data, which are lacking for most of the chemicals being tested currently for carcinogenicity by the National Toxicology Program, one should be careful not to become complacent regarding the firmness of (−) carcinogenicity assay results.

Roe (1987) has discussed the importance of the set of conditions selected for carcinogenicity assays and has suggested that "...apparent differences in response between different strains of rats (or different strains of mice) to the same chemical agent are more likely to be due to differences between the diets fed to the animals or to other differences in laboratory environments than to genetic differences between the strains."

IMPORTANCE OF REPLICATE EXPERIMENTS

One view of the rodent carcinogenicity assay is that the female mouse can be considered to replicate the male mouse; likewise, the female rat can be considered to replicate the male rat. This view considers that the species differences are greater than the sex differences. Another view, and the one to which we subscribe, is that the rodent carcinogenicity assay is four separate experiments, or four parts of one experiment, each with its own control, performed simultaneously. However, none of these four experiments is replicated, based on the generally accepted definition of a replicate experiment: an identical experimental protocol that is performed at another time, not simultaneously. An important difference between the set of conditions in STTs and animal carcinogenicity assays is that STT experiments are replicated, whereas carcinogenicity assays are generally not. Based on this consideration alone, we have greater confidence in a (+) or (−) call for an STT result than for a carcinogenicity assay result.

The main reason that people are forced into the uncomfortable position of accepting results from one unreplicated carcinogenicity assay as the "gold standard" is that experimentation under different sets of conditions is too expensive and lengthy to be generally feasible or practical. Thus, we are unlikely to obtain increased confidence in a given chemical's carcinogenicity or noncarcinogenicity under certain test conditions. In this regard, the reproducible genetic toxicity exhibited by many noncarcinogens (Shelby and Stasiewicz, 1984; Tennant et al., 1987; Waters et al., 1988a) should lead to a reconsideration of the firmness of the (−) rodent carcinogenicity results for these chemicals.

GENOTOXIC NONCARCINOGENS AND NONGENOTOXIC CARCINOGENS

A variety of genetic mechanisms has been implicated in carcinogenesis, and STTs have been developed that detect endpoints that are relevant to carcinogenesis (Ramel, 1986, 1988). Some of these endpoints include: (1) gene mutation (Bishop, 1987); (2) chromosomal aberrations (Duesberg, 1987); (3) aneuploidy or nondisjunction (Dellarco et al., 1986) and recombination (Wang et al., 1988), both of which may lead to homozygosity or hemizygosity of a recessive cancer gene (Cavenee et al., 1986); (4) recombination that can result in truncated cancer genes (Duesberg, 1987); (5) gene amplification (Fortner, 1987); and (6) mutation of mitochondrial DNA (Shay and Werbin, 1987).

Given this wide array of mechanisms, it may be premature to classify a carcinogen as nongenotoxic if it has not been examined for its ability to induce some of these endpoints. Heddle (1988) has argued further that a carcinogen might be declared nongenotoxic only if there is no evidence of genotoxicity or DNA damage *in vivo* in the tissue or cells in which the carcinogen is active. These considerations, combined with the use of standardized protocols and the uncertainties of the rodent carcinogenicity assay, complicate resolution of the issue of the prevalence of nongenotoxic carcinogens.

However, as pointed out previously, STTs identify genotoxicants, not carcinogens (Nestmann, 1986). Consistent with this is the observation by Ashby and Tennant (1988) and Ashby (1988) that STTs can be used to detect and assess the relative hazard of genotoxic carcinogens with relative ease. However, there are a number of carcinogens that, to the extent that they have been evaluated in STTs, are not genotoxic (Tennant et al., 1987). If these are actually carcinogenic, then (a) they may also be genotoxic, but they have not yet been evaluated under the appropriate conditions or at the appropriate endpoint; or (b) they really are nongenotoxic. As Trosko (1988) and Ashby (1988) have discussed, if this latter class of carcinogens actually exists, then new methods (and new thinking) will be required to detect and assess the relative hazard of nongenotoxic carcinogens. In this regard, Bridges (1986) has noted that if nongenotoxic carcinogens exist, then they cannot be used to evaluate the utility of STTs, which were designed specifically to detect genotoxic agents.

On the other hand, there are a number of noncarcinogens that show reproducible positive results in various STTs (Waters et al., 1988a). Because the carcinogenicity assay has not been replicated for most of these compounds, one must question the noncarcinogenicity of these compounds given their reproducible positive responses in STTs.

A reproducible biological response induced by a specific chemical in an STT whose endpoint is relatively well understood is a positive *genotoxic* response, even if the chemical is negative in a rodent carcinogenicity assay. Although it is common to refer to such a compound as a "false positive," we would draw the distinction between genotoxicity and carcinogenicity. The induction by a chemical of a reproducible biological response in a reasonably well understood STT is very real, reproducible biology. To declare such a result a "false positive" is to deny the validity (or even the reality) of the response in the STT and to evaluate the lack of response in the rodent carcinogenicity assay to an unjustified level of confidence.

UTILITY OF STTs FOR THE EVALUATION OF COMPLEX MIXTURES AND DETECTION OF ANTIMUTAGENS

People are exposed to mixtures of chemicals rather than to single chemicals (NRC, 1988). This fact alone illustrates the importance of complex environmental mixtures and, thus, of the need to study their potential health effects. Of all the areas of toxicology, genetic toxicology has been in the forefront of the study of complex mixtures (DeMarini, 1989; Lewtas, 1989). STTs have made it possible to evaluate the potential health effects of complex, environmental samples from air, water, soil, food, cigarettes, automobile exhaust, etc. Before the development of STTs, few studies of complex mixtures had been performed, and there was no systematic approach to evaluating the potential health effects of complex mixtures. These results from STTs have had a significant impact on our appreciation and understanding of the amount and types of mutagens present in our environment. As such, STT results with complex mixtures have been of enormous practical value in directing our attention to important environmental problems, such as diesel exhaust (Lewtas, 1982), cigarette smoke (DeMarini, 1983), and polluted drinking water (Loper, 1980).

Because of the chemical complexity of complex mixtures, it is difficult if not impossible to know *a priori* which chemicals to look for in a complex mixture. By chemically fractionating a complex mixture and testing the fractions for biological activity, one may use bioassays to identify the most biologically active fractions, which can then be chemically analyzed. This approach, which is called bioassay-directed chemical analysis, has been used most successfully with STTs to identify the primary mutagens in cigarette smoke (aromatic amines), diesel exhaust (nitro-aromatics), and urban air samples (polycyclic aromatic hydrocarbons). STTs have played a major role in making bioassay-directed chemical analysis a preferred approach to the study of complex mixtures.

STTs have also played a critical role in the development and application of the comparative potency approach to cancer risk assessment. This technique involves evaluating the tumorigenic and mutagenic potencies of complex mixtures in a variety of STTs, and then comparing the potencies to those of chemicals or mixtures for which human epidemiology has determined a cancer unit risk value. Such a comparison of the relative potencies permits an estimate of the cancer unit risk value for mixtures for which there would otherwise never be any human epidemiology (Albert et al., 1983; Lewtas et al., 1983). An example of this approach and its successful application has been reviewed recently for diesel exhaust by Nesnow (1989).

Because of the shortcomings of animal carcinogenicity assays and human epidemiology studies (Peter, 1982), and because of the central role of genotoxicity in the genesis of cancer and other disease, STTs have begun to be used extensively to identify antimutagens and potential anticarcinogens (Shankel et al., 1986). Pure compounds as well as complex mixtures (e.g., plant extracts) have been found to exhibit antimutagenic activities in a variety of STTs (Ames, 1983, 1986; Kada, 1984; Ramel et al., 1986; Shankel et al., 1986). These studies highlight the importance of STTs in detecting antimutagenic (as well as mutagenic) agents in the environment. In the absence of any other appropriate bioassays, STTs will continue to be essential for this purpose.

CONCLUSIONS

STTs detect genotoxic agents, not carcinogens specifically. However, there is sufficient evidence, based on mechanistic considerations alone, to say that genotoxic agents are potential carcinogens. Unlike animal carcinogenicity assays, STTs have high statistical power, are almost always replicated, can be performed rather easily under various sets of experimental conditions, are relatively inexpensive, and can detect a variety of endpoints relevant to cancer and other human diseases. The detection of genotoxic agents by means of STTs is important in its own right, quite apart from the detection of potential carcinogens.

Although STTs have proven invaluable for detecting genotoxic compounds, genotoxic complex mixtures, and antimutagens, they require additional development to overcome their many limitations. To this end, Clive (1988) has recommended further development of *in vivo* STTs, and Malling and Burkhart (1989) have recommended the development of transgenic mice that would permit the detection of genotoxic events in all tissues of the animal. The importance of mammalian cell assays has been emphasized by Green (1988), and the advantages and limitations of various mammalian cell specific-locus assays have been pointed out by DeMarini et al. (1989).

STTs are likely to continue to be refined and developed, resulting in STTs that are increasingly more relevant to human mutation and disease (Delehanty et al., 1986; Lohman et al., 1987). Their utility should not be judged solely against the questionable standard of a rodent carcinogenicity assay. We think that a prudent person would minimize his exposure to any agent shown to be genotoxic in replicated STTs, even if the agent is negative in a carcinogenicity assay.

ACKNOWLEDGEMENTS

H.E.B. acknowledges the support of the U.S. EPA Distinguished Visiting Scientist Program.

REFERENCES

ALBERT, R.E., LEWTAS, J., NESNOW, S., THORSLUND, T.W., ANDERSON, E. (1983). Comparative potency method for cancer risk assessment: Application to diesel particulate emissions. Risk Anal. 3:101–117.

AMES, B.N. (1983). Dietary carcinogens and anticarcinogens: Oxygen radicals and degenerative diseases. Science 221:1256–1264.

AMES, B.N. (1986). Overview: Food constituents as a source of mutagens, carcinogens, and anticarcinogens. In: Knudsen I (ed). "Genetic Toxicology of the Diet." New York: Alan R. Liss, pp. 3–22.

ASHBY, J. (1988). The separate identities of genotoxic and non-genotoxic carcinogens. Mutagenesis 3:365–366.

ASHBY, J., TENNANT, R.W. (1988). Chemical structure, Salmonella mutagenicity and extent of carcinogenicity as indicators of genotoxic carcinogenesis among 222 chemicals tested in rodents by the U.S. NCI/NTP. Mutat. Res. 204:17–115.

BISHOP, J.M. (1987). The molecular genetics of cancer. Science 235:305–311.

BRIDGES, B.A. (1986). Genetic toxicology at the cross-roads: A personal overview of the deployment of short-term tests. In: Montesano, R., Bartsch, H., Vainio, H., Wilbourn, J., Yamasaki, H. (eds). "Long-term and Short-term Assays for Carcinogens: A Critical Appraisal." Lyon, France: IARC Sci Publ No. 83, pp. 519–527.

BRIDGES, B.A. (1988). Genetic toxicology at the crossroads—a personal view on the deployment of short-term tests for predicting carcinogenicity. Mutat. Res. 205: 25–31.

BROCKMAN, H.E., DeMARINI, D.M. (1988). Utility of short-term tests for genetic toxicity in the aftermath of the NTP's analysis of 73 chemicals. Environ. Mol. Mutagen 11:421–435.

BRUSICK, D. (1983). Evaluation of chronic rodent bioassays and Ames assay tests as accurate models for predicting human carcinogens. In: Milman, H.A. and Sell, S. (eds). "Application of Biological Markers to Carcinogen Testing." New York: Plenum, pp. 153–163.

BRUSICK, D. (1988). Evolution of testing strategies for genetic toxicity. Mutat. Res. 205:69–78.

CAVENEE, W.K., KOUFOS, A., HANSEN, M.F. (1986). Recessive mutant genes predisposing to human cancer. Mutat. Res. 168:3–14.

CLAXTON, L.D., STEAD, A.G., WALSH, D. (1988). An analysis by chemical class of Salmonella mutagenicity tests as predictors of animal carcinogenicity. Mutat. Res. 205:197–225.

CLIVE, D. (1988). Genetic toxicology: can we design predictive in vivo assays? Mutat. Res. 205:313–330.

CROW, J.F. (1986). Population consequences of mutagenesis and antimutagenesis. In: Shankel, D.M., Hartman, P.E., Kada, T., Hollaender, A. (eds). "Antimutagenesis and Anticarcinogenesis Mechanisms." New York: Plenum, pp. 519–530.

DELEHANTY, J., WHITE, R.L., MENDELSOHN, M.L. (1986). Approaches to determining mutation rates in human DNA. Mutat. Res. 167:215–232.

DELLARCO, V.L., MAVOURNIN, K.H., WATERS, M.D. (1986). Aneuploidy data review committee: Summary compilation of chemical data base and evaluation of test methodology. Mutat. Res. 167:149–169.

DeMARINI, D.M. (1983). Genotoxicity of tobacco smoke and smoke condensate. Mutat. Res. 114:59–89.

DeMARINI, D.M. (1989). Environmental mutagens/complex mixtures. In: Li, A.P., Heflick, R.H. (eds). "Genetic Toxicology: a Treatise." Caldwell, NJ: Telford Press.

DeMARINI, D.M., BROCKMAN, H.E., DE SERRES, F.J., EVANS, H.H., STANKOWSKI, L.F., HSIE, A.W. (1989). Specific-locus mutations induced in eukaryotes (especially mammalian cells) by radiation and chemicals: A perspective. Mutat. Res., **220**:11–29.

DUESBERG, P.H. (1987). Cancer genes: Rare recombinants instead of activated oncogenes (a review). Proc. Natl. Acad. Sci. USA **84**:2117–2124.

FORTNER, J.G. (1987). "Accomplishments in Oncology: The Role of DNA Amplification in Tumor Initiation and Promotion." Philadelphia: Lippincott.

GARRETT, N.E., STACK, H.F., GROSS, M.R., WATERS, M.D. (1984). An analysis of the spectra of genetic activity produced by known or suspected human carcinogens. Mutat. Res. **134**:89–111.

GREEN, M.H.L. (1988). Short-term tests and the myth of the non-clastogenic mutagen. Mutagenesis **3**:369–371.

HARTMAN, P.E. (1983). Mutagens: Some possible health impacts beyond carcinogenesis. Environ. Mutagen. **5**:139–152.

HARTMAN, P.E., MORGAN, R.W. (1985). Mutagen-induced focal lesions as key factors in aging: a review. In: Sohal, R.S., Birnbaum, L.S., Cutler, R.G. (eds). "Molecular Biology of Aging: Gene Stability and Gene Expression." New York: Raven Press, pp. 93–136.

HASEMAN, J.K. (1983). Patterns of tumor incidence in two-year cancer bioassay feeding studies in Fischer 344 rats. Fund. Appl. Toxicol. **3**:1–9.

HEDDLE, J.A. (1988). Prediction of chemical carcinogenicity from *in vitro* genetic toxicity. Mutagenesis **3**:287–291.

HUFF, J.E., HASEMAN, J.K., BOORMAN, G.A., EUSTIS, S., MARONPOT, R.R., DeMARINI, D.M., PETERS, A., PERSHING, R., CHRISP, C., JACOBS, A.C. (1989). Pancarcinogenesis of benzene in Fischer rats and B6C3F$_1$ mice. Environ. Health Perspect., **82**, in press.

IARC (1982). IARC Monographs on the Evaluation of the Carcinogenic Risk of Chemicals to Humans, Suppl. 4, Chemicals, Industrial Processes and Industries Associated with Cancer in Humans, IARC Monographs, Volumes 1-29, Lyon, France: International Agency for Research on Cancer.

ICPEMC (1988). Testing for mutagens and carcinogens; the role of short-term genotoxicity assays. Mutat. Res. **205**:3–12.

KADA, T. (1984). Desmutagens and bio-antimutagens: Their action mechanisms and possible roles in the modulation of dose-mutation relationships. In: Tazima, Y. (ed). "Problems of Threshold in Chemical Mutagenesis." Mishima, Shizuoka, Japan: The Environmental Mutagen Society of Japan, pp. 73–82.

LEWTAS, J. (1982). "Toxicological Effects of Emissions from Diesel Engines." New York: Elsevier.

LEWTAS, J. (1989). Toxicology of complex mixtures of indoor air pollutants. Annu. Rev. Pharmacol. Toxicol., Vol. 29, in press.

LEWTAS, J., NESNOW, S., ALBERT, R.E. (1983). A comparative potency method for cancer risk assessment: Clarification of the rationale, theoretical basis, and application to diesel particulate emissions. Risk Anal. **3**:133–137.

LIJINSKY, W. (1988). Letter to the Editor. EMS Newsletter, January, pp. 6.

LOHMAN, P.H.M., VIJG, J., UITTERLINDEN, A.G., SLAGBOOM, P., GOSSEN, J.A., BERENDS, F. (1987). DNA methods for detecting and analyzing mutations in vivo. Mutat. Res. **181**:227–234.

LOPER, J.C. (1980). Mutagenic effects of organic compounds in drinking water. Mutat. Res. **76**:241–265.

MALLING, H.V., BURKHART, J.G. (1989). Use of ϕX174 as a shuttle vector for the study of *in vivo* mammalian mutagenesis. Mutat. Res., in press.

McCANN, J., AMES, B.N. (1976). Detection of carcinogens as mutagens in the *Salmonella/* microsome test: assay of 300 chemicals: Discussion. Proc. Natl. Acad. Sci. USA **73**:950–954.

McGREGOR, D. (1987). Letter to the Editor. EMS Newsletter, June, pp. 7.

MULLER, H.J. (1927). Artificial transmutation of the gene. Science **66**:84–87.

NESNOW, S. (1989). Mouse skin tumors as a predictor of human lung cancer for complex emissions: An overview. In: Slaga, T.J., Klein-Szanto, A.J.P., Boutwell, R.K., Stevenson, D.E., Spitzer, H.L., D'Motto, B. (eds). "Skin Carcinogenesis: Mechanisms and Human Relevance." New York: Alan R. Liss.

NESNOW, S., ARGUS, M., BERGMAN, H., CHU, K., FRITH, C., HELMES, T., McGAUGHY, R., RAY, V., SLAGA, T.J., TENNANT, R., WEISBURGER, E. (1987). Chemical carcinogens. A review and analysis of the literature of selected chemicals and the establishment of the Gene-Tox Carcinogen Data Base. Mutat. Res. **185**:1–195.

NESTMANN, E.R. (1986). A mutagen is a mutagen, not necessarily a carcinogen. In: Shankel, D.M., HARTMAN, P.E., KADA, T., HOLLAENDER, A. (eds). "Antimutagenesis and Anticarcinogenesis Mechanisms." New York: Plenum, pp. 423–424.

NRC (1988). "Complex Mixtures." Washington, DC: National Academy Press.

PENN, A., GARTE, S.J., WARREN, L., NESTA, D., MINDICH, B. (1986). Transforming gene in human atherosclerotic plaque DNA. Proc. Natl. Acad Sci. USA **83**:7951– 7955.

PETER, F.M. (1982). "Diet, Nutrition, and Cancer." Washington, DC: National Academy Press.

RAMEL, C. (1986). Deployment of short-term assays for the detection of carcinogens; genetic and molecular considerations. Mutat. Res. **168**:327–342.

RAMEL, C. (1988). Short-term testing—are we looking at wrong endpoints? Mutat. Res. **205**:13–24.

RAMEL, C., ALEKPEROV, U.K., AMES, B.N., KADA, T., WATTENBERG, L.W. (1986). Inhibitors of mutagenesis and their relevance to carcinogenesis: Report of ICPEMC Expert Group on Antimutagens and Desmutagens. Mutat. Res. **168**:47–65.

RAY, V.A., KIER, L.D., KANNAN, K.L., HAAS, R.T., AULETTA, A.E., WASSOM, J.S., NESNOW, S., WATERS, M.D. (1987). An approach to identifying specialized batteries of bioassays for specific classes of chemicals: Class analysis using mutagenicity and carcinogenicity relationships and phylogenetic concordance and discordance patterns. I. Composition and analysis of the overall data base. Mutat. Res. **185**:197–241.

ROE, F.J.C. (1987). Opinions on animal selection for the assessment of carcinogenicity. In: Roloff, M.V. (ed). "Human Risk Assessment. The Role of Animal Selection and Extrapolation." London: Taylor & Francis, pp. 31–44.

ROSENKRANZ, H.S. (ed). (1988). "Strategies for the Deployment of Batteries of Short-Term Tests." Special Issue of Mutat. Res., Vol. 205, Nos. 1–4.

SHANKEL, D.M., HARTMAN, P.E., KADA, T., HOLLAENDER, A. (1986). Antimutagenesis and Anticarcinogenesis Mechanisms. New York: Plenum.

SHAY, J.W., WERBIN, H. (1987). Are mitochondrial DNA mutations involved in the carcinogenic process? Mutat. Res. **186**:149–160.

SHELBY, M.D. (1988). The genetic toxicity of human carcinogens and its implications. Mutat. Res. **204**:3–15.

SHELBY, M.D., STASIEWICZ, S. (1984). Chemicals showing no evidence of carcinogenicity in long-term, two-species rodent studies: The need for short-term test data. Environ. Mutagen. **6**:871–878.

SOBELS, F.H. (1987). Environmental mutagenesis in retrospect. Mutat. Res. **181**:299–310.

SUGIMURA, T. (1988). Successful use of short-term tests for academic purposes: Their use in identification of new environmental carcinogens with possible risk for humans. Mutat. Res. **205**:33–39.

TENNANT, R.W., MARGOLIN, B.H., SHELBY, M.D., ZEIGER, E., HASEMAN, J.K., SPALDING, J., CASPARY, W., RESNICK, M., STASIEWICZ, S., ANDERSON, B., MINOR, R. (1987). Prediction of chemical carcinogenicity in rodents from in vitro genetic toxicity assays. Science **236**:933–941.

TROSKO, J.E. (1988). A failed paradigm: Carcinogenesis is more than mutagenesis. Mutagenesis **3**:363–366.

WANG, Y., MAHER, V.M.M., LISKAY, R.M., McCORMICK, J.J. (1988). Carcinogens can induce homologous recombination between duplicated chromosomal sequences in mouse L cells. Mol. Cell. Biol. **8**:196–202.

WATERS, M.D., BERGMAN, H.B., NESNOW, S. (1988a). The genetic toxicology of Gene-Tox non-carcinogens. Mutat. Res. **205**:139–182.

WATERS, M.D., STACK, H.F., BRADY, A.L., LOHMAN, P.H.M., HAROUN, L., VAINO, H. (1988b). Use of computerized data listings and activity profiles of genetic and related effects in the review of 195 compounds. Mutat. Res. **205**:295–312.

WILBOURN, J., HAROUN, L., HESELTINE, E., KALDOR, J., PARTENSKY, C., VAINIO, H. (1986). Response of experimental animals to human carcinogens: An analysis based upon the IARC Monographs programme. Carcinogenesis **7**:1853–1863.

ZEIGER, E. (1987). Carcinogenicity of mutagens: Predictive capability of the *Salmonella* mutagenesis assay for rodent carcinogenicity. Cancer Res. **47**:1287–1296.

SUBJECT INDEX

acetaminophen, 116–117
acetylcholinesterase, 113
actinomycin-D, 43
acute intoxications, 3
acute ocular, 137
acute poisoning, 4
acute toxicity, 6, 10
acute toxicity tests, 5
ADAPT SAR, 30
Alcian blue, 92
alkoxyacetic acid, 112
alternative methods, 11, 79, 81
alternative species, 167
alternative tests, 83
aminoglycoside antibiotics, 122
4-Aminosalicylic, 69
anesthetics, 167
animal bioassay, 16, 19
animal protectionists, 194
antivivisectionist groups, 4
approximate lethal doses, 4
aromatic amines, 211
ascitic mouse ovarian tumor cells, 90

Bayesian, 16
Bayesian statistics, 8
benz(e)aceanthrylene (B[e]A), 30
benzene, 209
benzo[a]pyrene (B[a]P), 30
Bhopal, 3
biliary dysfunction, 115
biological scaling, 48
biotransformation, 35, 115
bis(2-chloroethyl) sulfate, 167
blood-brain barrier, 113
brine shrimp (Artemia salina), 97
bromobenzene, 122
2-bromohydroquinone, 122
2-bromophenol, 122

cancer bioassay, 52

carbamates, 113
carbon tetrachloride, 116
carcinogenic, 15
carcinogenic potency, 22–23
carcinogenicity, 33, 61
carcinogenicity bioassay, 18, 20
Carcinogenicity Prediction and Battery
    Selection (CPBS) analysis, 16–17
CASE, 31
cefazolin, 121
cefoperazone, 121
ceftazidime, 121
cephaloglycin, 121
cephaloridine, 120–121
cephalothin, 120–121
chemical carcinogens, 206
chemotherapeutic agents, 42
chick embryo limb bud cells, 92
chick embryo neural crest cells, 92
chick embryo neural retina cell culture,
    93
chick embryos, 94
chlorinated aliphatics, 118
chloroform, 116
cholinesterase, 112
chromosomal damage, 15
cimetidine, 6
computer simulations, 38
concept of screens, 183
corrosion, 145
criteria for test evaluation, 176
cyclophosphamide, 80
cytotoxic response, 112
cytotoxicity, 122

decreased volume of test material, 167
desacetylation, 121
detoxification, 61
developmental toxicant screens, 80
developmental toxicity, 79
dichlorovinyl cysteine, 122

dicoumarol, 6
dimethyl sulfoxide, 167
Draize eye irritation, 61, 195
Draize Ocular Scoring Scale, 166, 169–171
Draize skin irritation, 61
Drosophila melanogaster, 94–96
Drosophila neuroblast-myoblast culture, 92

embryonal cell cultures, 103
embryonic organ cultures, 93
established cell lines, 87
ethylene dichloride, 46, 52
eye irritation, 138

fish embryos, 96

galactosamine, 117
genotoxic agents, 205
genotoxicity, 115
gentamicin, 122
germ-cell mutations, 206
glomerular epithelial cell, 120
glycol ethers, 112

haloalkanes, 118
hazard identification, 74
HeLa cell system, 112
hematopoietic system, 111
hepatocyte cultures, 117
hepatotoxicants, 118
hepatotoxicity, 116–119
HEPM assay, 90, 99
human carcinogens, 208
Hydra attenuata, 94–96
hydrofluoric, 146

in utero, 85–87
in vitro
    alternatives, 170
    assays, 81
    culture medium, 98
    cultures, 85
    methodologies, 42
    models, 178
    screen, 184
    teratogen, 104
    teratogen screens, 85–86
    teratogenicity assays, 103
    test, 90
    toxicology, 202
in vivo eye test, 177
intact embryos, 94
irritation, 145
irritation models, 64
isolated cell preparations, 42

kidney, 120

LD50, 4–8, 197
lethal dose 50%, 4
lidocaine, 40, 50
limit test, 9
lowest observable effect level (LOEL), 84

median lethal dose, 4
metabolic cooperation, 91
metabolites, 59, 74
methadone, 48
methotrexate, 43
methyl bromide, 167
methylene chloride, 45
microbial systems, 38
moderate irritation, 152
monkey, 40
monooxygenase system, 84
morbidity, 5
morphine, 48
mortality, 5
MOT assay, 90
mouse limb bud cells, 92
mutagenicity 33, 61–62
mutagenicity assay, 22
mutation, 15

neomycin, 122
nephrotoxicants, 125
nephrotoxicity, 120–123
neuroblastoma cell differentiation, 91
neurotoxicants, 112–113
n-hexane, 114
nitro-aromatics, 211
no observable effect level (NOEL), 84
nongenotoxic carcinogens, 207
nonhepatotoxicants, 118
norepinephrine, 44

ocular irritation, 147, 153, 182
ocular toxicities, 164
organophosphates, 113
other invertebrates, 97
ovarian tumors, 44

pain, 193
perchloroethylene, 46
peroxisome proliferation, 115
pharmacokinetic models, 39
pharmacokinetics, 38
pharmacological, 29
photosensitization, 145
phototoxicity, 145
phthalate esters, 112
physicochemical techniques, 38
physiological models, 4, 45
physiological pharmacokinetic models, 40
plasticizers, 146
polychlorinated biphenyls, 45
polycyclic aromatic hydrocarbons (PAH's), 30, 211
poxvirus proliferation test, 91
primary cultures of embryonal cells, 91
primary dermal irritation (PDI), 168, 184
prioritization, 59
proximal tubule, 122
proximal tubule cell, 120
psychotherapeutic agents, 114

putative metabolites, 61

rabbit eye irritation, 64, 161–164
rabbit skin irritation, 63
rat embryo cultures, 85
rat hepatocytes, 85
rat midbrain and hind limb bud cell culture, 93
rat oral LD50, 61–64
risk assessment, 61
rodent embryo culture, 97

sensitization, 145
severe irritation or corrosion, 152
skin irritation, 63, 169
somatic mutations, 205
staggered eye irritation test, 184
streptomycin D_{37}, 122
structural modifications, 59, 74
structure-activity relationships (SAR), 29–30, 60
STTs, 208, 212
substantial irritation, 152
systemic toxicity, 10

teratogen screens, 80
teratogenicity assays, 79
therapeutic indexes, 6
thymidine, 92
tissue culture methodologies, 38
tissue homogenates, 42
TOPKAT program, 61, 69, 76
toxicological, 29
toxicological screening, 7
trichloroethylene, 116

use of prescreens, 168

whole embryo, 103

Xenopus embryos, 95
Xenopus laevis, 95